THE DOLCE DIET
LIVING LEAN

MIKE DOLCE

Conrad James Books
Las Vegas, NV
www.conradjamesbooks.com

Printed in the United States of America.

ISBN 978-0-615-53167-0

Conrad James Books
conradjamesbooks.com

Edited by Brandy Roon & Sarah Veit
Cover & Interior Design by Jun Hanawa
Photos: Tom Hill Photos, TomHillPhotos.com

"Wisdom is not a product of schooling but of the lifelong attempt to acquire it."
—*Albert Einstein*

CONTENTS

INTRODUCTION

Living Lean is an easily adapted approach to enhancing your health and wellness while leading a busy life. I'm not going to waste your time with hundreds of pages dedicated to terminology and definitions in an attempt to prove validity while hiding behind science. It's not necessary.

I simply tell you what works.

It amazes me how many diet plans are thrust onto the market each year that claim they're going to save the world - that is, until the next plan comes out. The people who swear by a diet today may lose 40 lbs. in a month, but three months from now, most will have gained it back and then some. Just take a look around.

The title of this book is *The Dolce Diet: Living Lean*, but this is not a diet.

Living Lean promotes a healthy lifestyle based on the practices and principles of longevity science that I use with today's top athletes. I won't advise you to drive yourself crazy counting every single calorie, nor will I advise you to universally exclude healthy food groups you already enjoy.

Here's why: Those techniques don't work.

But wait, you might say. Those techniques *do* work. What if I consume fewer calories than I expend? Won't I lose weight? Or, what if I stop eating all grains? I'll lose weight then, right?

You may lose weight for a few days, maybe even a few weeks, but soon enough the large majority of us simply cannot sustain that type of deprivation and eventually fall off the fad diet wagon.

Living Lean is proudly based on ideals derived from my personal experiences, observations and continued results with the world's most recognized athletes. I'm thrilled to share them here, so you can immediately begin leading a healthier life at your own pace - one positive choice at a time.

THE DOLCE DIET
LIVING LEAN

MIKE DOLCE

CHAPTER ONE

BAPTISM

"There are two mistakes one can make along the road to truth...not going all the way, and not starting."
—*Hindu Prince Gautama Siddharta*

The steam in the bathroom was so thick it was hard to see what was happening. I blinked. Yes, this was real. A baptism was about to take place. The bedroom was pushing 95 degrees. Christian music pumped through the sound system, and there was a constant parade of smiling faces popping in to say hi.

The athlete was submerged to his chest in a steaming bath with lavender-eucalyptus bubbles floating like swans all around him.

Words were spoken that I couldn't quite hear. I didn't have to. The fighter was rejoicing. He'd already lost 30 lbs. during training camp and today had to lose just eight more. In this situation, some people would look like they were suffering. But as the priest made the sign of the cross over the fighter's head, he beamed the smile of a young boy. This wasn't just a weight cut. This was a spiritual moment during which I couldn't help but think: How did I get here?

Weight has been my main focus for more than twenty years; as a competitor, as a coach and as a consultant.

I purposely drove my body weight to 280 lbs. as powerlifter to achieve my goal of squatting over 800 lbs. Three years later, I set the record for fastest knockout in the International Fight League while competing as a 170 lb. mixed martial artist. I lost 110 lbs. while maintaining a vibrant level of health and vitality.

Now, as a peak performance coach, I continue to develop these methods while working with the most elite athletes in mixed martial arts. I'd like to share them here with you.

THIRD GRADE

It was the end of a typical school day for me. I could hear the pounding of waves on the beach a few blocks away as I made my way home from school. I tossed my backpack on the dining room chair and headed straight for the refrigerator. That's when I noticed the prevailing silence. In a house with four kids, silence is rare.

The backdoor was open, but the screen door was shut. I could see my mother in the yard hustling toward the stairs, toward me. All I could think was, Uh, oh. What did I do?

"Hold your father," she yelled.

That's when I saw my dad sitting on the back stairs, tilting awkwardly to the side, incoherent. The minutes that followed were a blur of emergency sirens, color and people. Our next door neighbor was a police officer and the first emergency responder on the scene. Then came the ambulance and the craziness. Neighbors from up and down 8th Avenue flooded our driveway offering support, but mostly asking what had happened. I didn't know. But later, I found out my father suffered a stroke.

I was nine.

A stroke is caused by the rupturing or the blockage of an artery. This prevents part of the brain from receiving oxygen, and in minutes, brain cells begin to die, resulting in brain damage, disability and death. Studies show up to 80 percent of strokes can be prevented simply by reducing risk.

My father was a first generation Italian immigrant who began smoking cigarettes before he was a teenager and continued to do so for nearly twenty years before he quit. He remained smoke-free for another twenty years before his stroke.

Cigarette smoking is a leading cause of stroke along with high blood pressure, high cholesterol and diabetes – conditions that are predominantly influenced by lifestyle; notably poor diet and lack of exercise. Not surprisingly, these same conditions are the leading causes of heart disease and obesity.

My father looked like he was in great shape. But his insides were a different story. He cooked with butter, ate fried foods regularly, and usually unwound with a few beers at night. He routinely skipped breakfast, but always grabbed a Thermos full of coffee before he left the house.

His sixty-hour work schedule kept him away from meaningful exercise and increased his level of stress. He was a solid provider and an excellent father. He always took great care of us, but in turn, he did not take care of himself.

A few months after the stroke, my mother and I stopped by the local 7-Eleven for a gallon of whole milk and a loaf of Wonder bread. Like most kids would do, I began scanning the shelves for a candy bar, but my eyes caught on something else. I remember the moment perfectly. Instead of the candy bar, I reached for a magazine with Conan the Barbarian on the cover. Only he wasn't dressed like Conan. He was standing on the beach surrounded by a pile of weights and throngs of women. I forgot all about the candy bar and asked my mom to buy me the magazine, which she did, surprisingly without arguing. That was my first conscious decision in which I put my health first.

That night, I didn't sleep. There were pictures of Franco Colombu deadlifting nearly 700 lbs. There were pictures of Frank Zane looking as near perfect as a human could. And later, guys like Dorian Yates with his sheer muscularity and physical presence. There were hundreds, maybe thousands, of athletes just like them whom I studied.

What did they eat?

How did they train?

And how could I do that, too?

In short time, I was lecturing my mother on the saturated fat content of whole milk and why she should be feeding us plain chicken breast instead of bulk ground beef. Every day, I learned something new. Even then, I felt it was my obligation to share this knowledge. Don't get me wrong. A lot of the things I read in these magazines didn't make sense even to my young brain, but I still recognized salesmanship and gluttony over scientific fact and applicable health benefits.

My enthusiasm wasn't confined to nutrition or lecturing family members. The house I grew up in was built in the early 1900's and the windows were outfitted with weights that acted as counterbalances when the windows were opened or closed. One day, while playing in the basement, I discovered a set of these weights. I immediately assumed they were dumbbells, and I'd spend hours with my magazines opened to articles detailing the workouts done by my favorite athletes. I performed every exercise hundreds of times for thousands of reps. No doubt I was extremely over-trained! (I wouldn't learn the principles of periodization and central nervous system recovery for a few more years.)

FRESHMAN YEAR

It was the spring before high school. I was five-foot-four and maybe just over 100 lbs. I was working at a local athletic store scrubbing silk screens at a chemical tub of all things. A few doors down was a hardcore bodybuilding gym called The Muscle Shop. I wanted a membership there, but the age of consent was fifteen with a parent's signature. I was thirteen.

Driven by the need to know what happened inside those walls, I did what any desperate boy would do in my situation. I lied.

It took me a couple days to build up the courage to walk through the big wooden door. And when I finally did I felt like I'd fallen through the proverbial rabbit hole. This was a whole new world of which I couldn't wait to become a citizen. Metallica blasted from mounted, dust-coated speakers in a cement room bursting with thousands of pounds of weights, barbells and steel cages. And then there were these massive, mostly ugly monsters walking around in clown clothes.

There wasn't an office. Only a stool, a shelf, and a cash register. After a few minutes of me standing there looking like I'd seen the Second Coming, this short, stocky guy with eyebrows as big as his mustache walked toward me. I froze. He looked exactly like Dennis Tinerino, whom most of you might not recognize as Mr. America 1967, but I sure did. I'd read dozens of articles about him, but as the guy got closer, the mirage faded.

This was Joe, the owner. He had a great build. All his muscles were perfectly rounded and they fit together flawlessly. He was wearing an orange tank top he'd obviously tailored to show off more skin than the original designer intended. He introduced himself and – seeing how scrawny I was – promptly told me I had to be fifteen to sign up.

It was $99 for three months, but there was a catch. I had to convince my mother to sign the consent papers. I ran out of there, grabbed my bike and pedaled fast. Would she be cool with this? I was about to find out.

Dropping the bike on our front lawn, I bolted into the house. Mom was scraping dinner together and barely glanced at me as I started rambling.

"Okay," she said, cutting me off mid-sentence.

She didn't ask anything about age, and I certainly wasn't going to tell her. Mom went back to cooking while I stared at her expectantly. She glanced up.

"Can we go now?" I asked.

She wasn't thrilled, but didn't say no as she put away dinner and grabbed her purse. I followed her out the door.

I had the money to pay for it. Money wasn't the issue. I had coffee cans filled with $5 bills from the athletic shop and a newspaper route so the enrollment fee was of no consequence.

We walked into the gym and it was the same crazy zoo scene from before. I noticed more people looking this way now that I was standing there with my mother. She was the only woman in the gym.

Joe came over and told her what he'd told me earlier, only this time much more politely. During his sales pitch he'd told her he'd put me on a fitness program and that he'd teach me everything I needed to know to get started. Sounded great to me!

She signed the consent form. The deal was done. I asked my mom if I could stay and get started. She had no problem with it, but how was I going to get home? I told her I'd walk. It was about three miles to my house. Yeah, I was that excited. We parted ways, and I walked back into the gym.

I was standing by the register trying to make eye contact with Joe, who was talking to some guys sitting on weight benches. They looked like they were training, but after ten minutes of watching them, they hadn't done anything. (Today, that's a habit of gym-goers that absolutely drives me crazy. Don't monopolize the gym equipment. Get in, get out, get it done.)

Joe finally noticed me. He came over looking slightly peeved. I'd guessed the story he'd been telling was a whopper. He asked if I forgot something.

"No," I said. "I want to start training."

Now his look was more of disappointment than annoyance. His face went blank for a second.

"Follow me," he said.

He brought me over to a steel contraption of pulleys and weights with six different stations. Joe told me to go to each station, do ten reps and move on to the next. Go around the circuit three times, he'd said. He pointed me to the Triceps Pressdown and showed me how to do that for two or three reps.

"There ya go," he said as he walked away.

It was the last time I ever talked to that guy.

The steel V-bar in my hands was attached to a 200 lb. stack of weights. Although I was only using 40 of those pounds, I felt invincible! I could feel my body merge with the steel during each repetition. It became more like a team effort; my body, my mind and the weight stack. I was hooked.

From that first set, I knew exactly how to train myself, how to pair muscle groups, increase strength in specific areas of my choosing, lose weight, or increase endurance. I was a natural. I put on 40 lbs. of muscle that year. I began high school as a 114 lb. skinny kid and came back sophomore year at a solid 154. I was still only five-foot-four.

All the local cops trained at my gym, and I was lifting more than they were. At fifteen, I thought that was something to be pretty proud of considering I focused on the hardest lifts that most others naturally avoided. While they were performing leg extensions and biceps curls, I was straining at the squat rack or performing weighted chin-ups.

I made the varsity wrestling team as a freshman, having never wrestled a single match in my life. I walked onto the mat the first day of tryouts and pinned my opponent in twenty seconds with a move that doesn't even exist. I pretty much just manhandled him. Somehow I wrapped his knees around his head and held him there until the coach slapped the mat and shouted, "Pin!"

When I got up the assistant coach came over. He was a well-known college wrestler from our area with a grizzled face, ugly ears and a wad of chewing tobacco nesting in his upper lip.

"Have you ever wrestled before?"

Embarrassed, I shook my head and said, "No."

He smiled. "I didn't think so, but you made the team."

When formal practice started, the coaches immediately moved me out of the freshman group and into the sophomore group, and then to the juniors and, finally, the seniors. By the second week, I was working out with the varsity squad and doing pretty damn well.

The night before our first match, the coaches sat us around the mat to give us a pep talk. They finished by saying they'd chosen four captains: Two seniors, a junior, and me.

When I returned sophomore year, my teammates noticed the big difference in my appearance. They were amazed at how much stronger I was than everybody else and how I would never get tired.

They wanted to make the same physical gains. So I helped them. To repay me, some guys would drive me to practice or pay for my lunch, and I'd show them how to lift weights, eat properly, and take them on runs.

I'd design my teammates' weight cuts and rehydration for same-day wrestling matches or multi-day tournaments. Back then I was relying on performance-science tempered with my own experience of gaining or losing up to 20 lbs. three times a week.

This pursuit became my obsession. I poured through countless books, magazines, research journals and abstracts as well as attended seminars, conferences and more classes than I can remember.

Clearly, this remains my obsession, and I have continued to evolve my work around the principles of longevity science, realizing that life extends far past an athlete's career.

CHAPTER TWO

HELP IS NOT A FOUR-LETTER WORD

"Example isn't another way to teach, it is the only way to teach."
—*Albert Einstein*

As I'm writing this, someone in Slovakia just bought my weight-cut manual, *The Dolce Diet: 3 Weeks to Shredded.* That modest publication has sold in more than 85 countries worldwide. It is the cornerstone of a nutritional philosophy that's helped thousands of average men and women annihilate countless pounds and keep it off.

I'm grateful so many people put their faith in me – people like Justin B. from Philadelphia, Pa., who lost more than 170 lbs., or Anderson W. from Loveland, Ohio, who lost more than 65 lbs. I am humbled and blessed, and I'm always happy to help others.

It's not easy to ask for help.

Many people misconstrue asking for help as a weakness, but I believe that admitting when we need help is a great strength and a testament to our character. Humility and an open mind go a long way in life and do much to increase our self-worth. Sometimes help can take the form of a challenge to which we must rise.

In high school, Derrick Dorfman was this shy kid with white-blond hair and light blue eyes. He was skinnier – and nicer – than anyone else I knew. He sat next to me in most every class, since we were assigned seats alphabetically by last name.

Derrick and I started off the same as freshmen – skinny. I came back sophomore year more muscular and looking like a senior, having gained 40 lbs. that summer. Derrick, who still sat next to me, might've lost a pound.

My conversations with my friends would often be about girls – and girls. But Derrick would always ask me about working out and eating: How do I train?

What's a bench press? What's a squat?

I decided to invite him to the school wrestling room after classes one day. I showed him the squat, the bench press and the deadlift. The first day he looked like a baby horse straining to pick up an oak tree with no balance, hardly any strength, and no real concept of physical exertion.

By the third time I brought him to the wrestling room, his form was nearly perfect. And we had 5 lb. plates on the bar. Derrick was on his way. Junior year, Derrick took his seat beside me with the confidence of a man.

Thirty pounds of added muscle will do that to a guy.

HIGH SCHOOL WRESTLING

Between my junior and senior years, I attended a wrestling camp run by Iowa Hawkeyes coach Dan Gable, who is arguably the most famous American wrestler of all time. What I gleaned from the top wrestling camp in the nation motivated me in several ways.

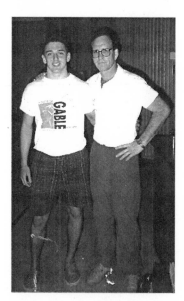

Mike, 16, weighing 160 lbs. with coach Dan Gable.

For instance, they had trainers working on the side of the mat to immediately diagnose any strain, rip or tear. This propelled me to learn everything I could about injury prevention. I constantly questioned the trainers and even sat with them at lunch to pick their brains. I had always focused on pushing the boundaries of bigger, stronger, faster, but not until Camp Gable did I realize the importance of solidifying the infrastructure. I had no idea injury prevention and rehabilitation could play such a dramatic role in sports performance.

Looking back now I shouldn't have been nearly as surprised when I received a pamphlet called "The College Wrestler's Diet" as part of my welcome kit. Actually, surprised isn't the right word. Aghast is more fitting. The top wrestlers in the country were relying on pseudo bodybuilding meal plans and calorie deficit techniques mixed with severe dehydration and over-exertion while attempting to perform at a world-class level. Noting this, confidence in my own methods grew. Seeing such high caliber athletes operate at a nutritional deficit compelled me to learn more about using food as a fuel to build the body, not tear it down.

There's no doubt that the work ethic I adopted from Camp Gable is a benefit I'll forever retain. I've used Iowa's example to set my own in every training camp I'm part of. I often train right alongside my athlete. I eat what he eats, sleep when he sleeps and always wake before he does to begin organizing our day. Why? To set a positive example, a goal to which I constantly strive. Working hard for a cause you believe in is the most rewarding of all tasks. It costs nothing yet reaps so much in return.

SENIOR YEAR

My wrestling team had just lost a match – badly. Coach was angry to say the least. The following day we knew what was coming. We always had a punishment if we lost. I was the only guy to win during the match. I still remember I won by a throw to a pin. Coach excused me from punishment, which turned out to be push-ups. But two things made me join in on the punishment despite receiving immunity: First, I was a team captain, and second, I didn't want my teammates calling me a wimp!

After hundreds of push-ups, and other grueling exercises of physical torture, guys were having problems lifting their bodies off the floor. Everyone was dropping into pools of their own sweat.

Finally, and to our horror, Coach demanded everyone hold the last push-up for as long as we could. Half the team dropped immediately. The other half stayed up. Not surprising, the half that continued on were mostly the guys on varsity. They actually pushed until their arms shook, bodies convulsed, pain distorted their faces, knees touched the floor, and then finally they collapsed through sheer exhaustion.

Each guy who collapsed meant I was one step closer to being done. There was no way I was going to quit before anyone else. I was the only one who didn't have to do it, and I was going to do it the best. As the last guy fell, I looked up and saw a freshman still posted in his push-up position. Darin Jacobs.

He was a skinny, blonde wiseass freshman, and he was all the way on the other side of the mat grimacing in pain like his feet were on fire, but he was staring straight through me.

We bonded right there. I both hated and loved him at the same time because as each guy hit the floor, my anticipation of being able to stop increased. And boy was I ready to stop at this point. But then I knew Darin was waiting for me to drop so he could be the last one standing. Now the situation was worse than if I'd just quit before while some of the other seniors were still in the game. Letting a freshman beat me would be the story of the day in school tomorrow, and immediately I had full energy.

I stared right back at Darin. I saw his arms start to quiver, his chest shake and his face contort hideously. Darin collapsed. I gave it a few more seconds for punctuation and, instead of falling, got to my feet and jogged around the wrestling room. The rest of the team followed.

I'd learned something that day. Our greatest selves emerge from our greatest challenges. That, and never underestimate the little guy. I gave Darin a ride home from practice that day. We've been friends ever since. Oh, and we won our next match.

CHAPTER THREE

GETTING IT WRONG IS HOW I GOT IT RIGHT

"We learn wisdom from failure much more than from success. We often discover what will do, by finding out what will not do..."
—Samuel Smiles

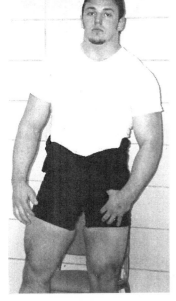

Mike, 19, competing at a powerlifting competition at 210 lbs.

I ended up graduating high school at 210 lbs. of solid muscle. I'd received a college scholarship for wrestling but subsequently blew out my shoulder, so there went the scholarship. I didn't want to stop competing, but where does a grown man wrestle besides the WWE? Though I do enjoy some good *wrasslin'* that lifestyle simply wasn't an option.

Maybe it was time to switch sports.

The Muscle Shop was more of a bodybuilder's gym. After a few years, that style of training - the slow, smooth sculpting - was not for me. During that time, I gained a considerable amount of lean muscle mass and mastered the technical aspects specific to bodybuilding methodology, but I needed something new. My junior year in high school I switched to a powerlifting gym a few towns over.

I talked a couple of buddies into joining my new gym, and we became a little crew. We kept each other accountable to show up on time and talk enough trash to push each other forward.

Friday night was our squat night. While everybody else was getting ready to go out for a night on the town, we eagerly seized the opportunity of an empty gym. I could think of no better way to spend my Friday nights.

There were three power racks in the gym, only one of which was truly hardcore. It was the main stage and had the best stories attached to it. This is where we always squatted.

That night, there were two guys in the rack we didn't know personally, but they were legends in the gym. We got there just as they were starting their own squat workout, but they invited us to jump in. So we did.

They were the two strongest guys in the gym and at least ten years older than us. For the last five years, they'd been setting records in all of the major powerlifting and strongman organizations. We lifted together from then on, and I began my internship to a new style of training. Within six months of that first workout I competed in the 181 lb. weight-class, cutting down from my normal body weight of 198. I squatted 525 lbs. and set a teenage record.

I was seventeen.

For ten years, I was schooled in the ways of powerlifting, which is so much more than pushing heavy weights around. There are several factors to consider such as periodization, volume, intensity, speed, strength and elasticity.

SUPER-SIZED

Later in my powerlifting career I'd squatted 710 lbs. in the 242 lb. weight-class while weighing 238 lbs. That night, I turned to my girlfriend and said, "What do you think about me moving up to the 275 lb. class and going for an 800?"

Brandy, who's now my wife, looked at me with a perfect poker face and said very supportively, "You have to promise me when you're done, you'll drop back down to 200 lbs."

When we first met three years prior, I weighed 198 lbs. and was built just like Superman. She's seen quite the metamorphosis. Looking back, I can't imagine how I would have reacted if she told me that she had wanted to gain another 40 lbs. on top of the roughly forty or so pounds gained since we first met.

What can I say?

That evening, I came up with a plan of action. To truly commit to my goal, I had to set a completion date. I gave myself nine months. My training system was pretty darn effective, so I didn't need to recreate the wheel here, just continually evolve my methods with an open mind. My goal of weighing 275 lbs. sounded like a fun one (yes, I got to eat more!), but as a dedicated athlete, I was eating only as a means to improve my leverage points and increase skeletal density, enabling me to safely handle heavier weights.

Over the past few years, I had already bumped my natural weight up about 60 lbs. and for me to add another 40 lbs. in a functional manner meant I needed a lot more nutrients.

While researching, I picked up an old magazine and opened to an article written by bench-press phenom J.M. Blakely. The topic was eating to gain weight.

"If you want to beat the man, you've got to out-eat the man!" he wrote.

And, that's what I did. I began eating. Well, it was more like gorging: Eight, whole-egg omelets with half a loaf of bread, a half-gallon of whole milk and a few bananas for breakfast. For lunch, I'd order a double dinner portion of penne chicken in vodka sauce, a cheeseburger, French fries and an entire loaf of garlic bread with double cheese, two cans of Dr. Pepper and a quart of whole milk.

For dinner, I would go anywhere that sounded good between my office and my house and eat more food than a family of four. To top it all off, I would end my night with an entire pepperoni pizza that I would cover with another half-pound of provolone slices, a half-gallon of Breyer's chocolate ice cream and a king-sized Snickers bar.

The first month went pretty slow, but after four weeks, I weighed 248 lbs. I'd gained 10 lbs. and was handling heavier weights. I thought I was off to a good start.

For another two weeks, the scale didn't change and a few times my weight even dropped, though my calories didn't. I became so obsessed that I would actually weigh myself after each meal, desperately trying to break the 250 lb. barrier.

Finally, my weight shot from 247 lbs. to 254 lbs. in two days. From then on, there wasn't a single day I didn't gain weight. Before I knew it, I was 280 lbs. and starting to train for my 800 lb. squat attempt.

This was the most uncomfortable point in my life.

Everything I did revolved around weight – body weight, barbell weight or the weight of the massive amounts of food I needed to fuel my training sessions.

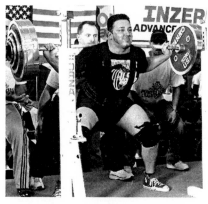

Mike, 280 lbs., competes as a super heavyweight powerlifter.

In my younger years, I thought this was glamorous. Looking back now, I know I was a complete idiot! I was exhausted twenty-two hours of the day. The only time I felt energized were the two hours I spent in the gym. Every other moment inside my skin was horror.

I developed a severe case of sleep apnea from my own body mass crushing my ability to breathe. My resting heart rate shot up from the mid-60's to the mid-80's. I constantly sweated and had to bring "back-up" shirts with me wherever I went because I would sweat through my original shirt by day's end.

But, boy was I powerful. So powerful in fact, that I blew past my intended goal of 800 lbs. and wound up squatting 840 lbs. Mission accomplished! But my health was the collateral damage.

I made an appointment with my family doctor, whom I hadn't visited in maybe three years. I walked in for a simple physical and walked out hooked to a Holter monitor. In a ten-minute appointment I felt like I had aged twenty years. Although in my mid-twenties, I was discussing elevated cholesterol, dangerously high blood pressure, irregular heart beat and sleep apnea, conditions much more common with the forty-five and older crowd.

Scared for my well-being, I immediately turned my focus to longevity nutrition and was blessed to work with some of the most brilliant minds in the field of life extension and disease management.

Today, I walk around at just about 192 lbs. at 7 percent body fat. Ironically, I'm actually a more powerful athlete now. I can squat 500 lbs. with no belt or knee wraps for 20 full reps, and I can run 10 miles any day of the week. My resting heart rate hovers in the low 40's, and I can easily maintain a heart rate above 170 beats per minute for hours on end. Due to my bi-yearly checkups and complete blood tests, I know that all my primary indicators of health are at or above perfect.

The reason for such improved numbers was my emphasis on longevity science. Learning firsthand the negative effects performance nutrition can have on the human body, I became an advocate of whole foods.

For the past ten years, The Dolce Diet has been evolving as a longevity program, which has been proven successfully at the highest levels of mixed martial arts. What makes my methods unique is that they are equally employed by those seeking to extend general health and wellness.

THE MOVE TO MMA

The health risks of powerlifting and the demands I put my body through had a definite role in prompting me to shift my focus toward mixed martial arts. I had already been coaching many East Coast mixed martial artists and jiu jitsu competitors as well as my stable of wrestlers. In order to be a better coach in this growing sport, I decided to start grappling.

The first mixed martial arts class I took was at a local Renzo Gracie affiliate in Neptune, N.J. I was 256 lbs.

Leaner, faster, stronger – I wanted to be all those adjectives once again, like I was in high school. Except now, the emphasis also was on being healthier.

A year later, I signed up for a three-day camp to be held at Team Quest in Portland, Ore., which was widely considered the top MMA fight team in the world. Randy Couture had just beaten Tito Ortiz, Chuck Liddell and Vitor Belfort to retain the UFC Light Heavyweight world title. This was where he trained, along with twenty other of the top professional fighters in the world.

I trained hard leading up to the camp and felt the same nervous excitement I did before I went to Camp Gable. I envisioned the same grueling practices and wanted to be prepared.

The camp came and went. It was an eye opening experience. The guys were just as tough as I expected and the techniques being taught were certainly world-class.

Again, I was surprised to learn that the areas most overlooked were strength, conditioning and nutrition. I spent much of my time in Oregon speaking at length with the coaches and athletes on these topics. I learned and taught quite a bit, and best of all I made friends there, a few of which I've kept till this day.

A week after settling back into my regular life, the phone rang. It was the head coach of Team Quest. After exchanging pleasantries he came straight out and asked me if I would consider moving across the country to be a part of the team.

Silence.

I pulled the phone from my ear and stared at it a minute. I was working in an office wearing a suit and tie with a fully vested 401K plan and six weeks of paid vacation. Now, the opportunity to leave all that and take a chance at a guaranteed nothing had just come calling. I politely thanked the coach for the opportunity and asked for a few days to think about it.

Later that day, I sat in a board meeting and looked around the table. I was twenty years younger than my closest peer. Most of them were overweight. They were all nice guys in their own right, but they just seemed so damned stressed out with work, with family, and with social standing. Most of the conversation was about paying bills or going to the bar. And that's when I knew I had to get out of there.

That night, I took Brandy – still my girlfriend - out to dinner and told her about my offer to move away. I braced myself for what I thought she would say and she surprised me once again.

"Michael, you have to do this."

This wasn't only a sacrifice for me. This was a sacrifice for her also. She had worked very hard since college building a strong résumé and had achieved a dream job as a journalist. We could always come back to New Jersey and try to pick up where we left off, but we both agreed that if we didn't do this, we'd regret it.

That's when I proposed to her. We were married four weeks later and spent our honeymoon driving across the country to start our new life together.

CHAPTER FOUR

3 WEEKS TO SHREDDED

"Call me a braggart, call me arrogant. People at ABC (and elsewhere) have called me worse. But when you need the job done on deadline, you'll call me."
—Sam Donaldson

Gresham, Ore., is rarely sunny and today wasn't any different. I pulled the keys from the ignition and grabbed my training gear for team practice. The dirt parking lot was still muddy from the ongoing downpours infamous in the Pacific Northwest. I heard footsteps and turned to see my coach squishing across the lot toward me.

"What do you weigh?" he said.

"192," I lied, anticipating what he'd say next.

He didn't break his stride as he walked past me and got into his truck.

"You make 170?"

I nodded. "No problem."

He slammed the door and drove off.

I actually weighed 207 lbs.

Chris Wilson was the starting welterweight on the Portland Wolfpack, a team in the newly founded International Fight League (IFL). The IFL was built around a team concept. Each team, headed by an MMA legend, comprised five guys in five weight classes – lightweight, welterweight, middleweight, light heavyweight and heavyweight.

A spot on the team meant a monthly salary, health benefits and a very respectable purse with win incentives to each of the rostered athletes. It was the corner office job in our profession.

Being close friends with Chris, I knew he was fielding offers from other organizations as his unorthodox Muay Thai style quickly made him a fan favorite and a fearsome opponent. I deduced that a good offer had come in and his welterweight spot for the Wolfpack's next fight needed to be filled.

I hadn't weighed less than 184 lbs. since junior year in high school, but I didn't care. After just one pro fight as a middleweight I was ready to take another step. The notion of employing my skills as a performance coach excited me much more than the paycheck I would receive as an athlete.

There would be no point of making the weight just to look like crap and get beat up on national TV. I had to make sure that I was in the best shape of my life. And I was.

I'd lost 38 lbs. in four weeks and weighed in at 169 lbs. for my IFL debut. The next night, I knocked out my opponent in 19 seconds and set the record for the fastest KO in the organization's history, and clinched the win for my team.

As an athlete, I'd done my job that night. But as a coach, I'd set a new standard. Guiding an athlete's weight cut is like guiding a ship in to dock. If the wind is off or the navigation is deciphered incorrectly it's easy to sail off course.

I cut to 170 lbs. repeatedly over the next two years. During that time, my stable of UFC athletes continued to grow, and the students in my newly established Women's FIT program continually watched me shrink from over 200 lbs. to 170 lbs. in the course of a few weeks. They wanted to know what magic formula I used. I kept telling them it's not magic, it's common sense.

Finally, my wife suggested we sit down and write a description of one of my cuts. She typed it up and we called it *The Dolce Diet: 3 Weeks to Shredded.* We got it printed, and I gave it to my students who then gave it to their friends and so on.

And then the results started rolling in. Office workers, housewives, nurses, teachers, factory workers; these were all non-athletes who experienced life-changing weight loss based on one of my weight cuts. I felt so blessed to be able to share this knowledge with people who were truly benefitting from it.

Today, *3 Weeks to Shredded* continues to garner the acclaim of everyday people who are losing weight smartly and keeping it off.

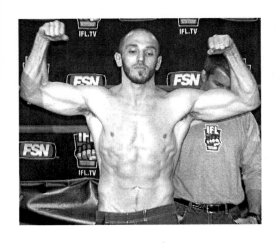

Mike loses 110 lbs. to compete as a professional mixed martial artist. Here, he weighed in at 169 lbs. the day before he set the record for the fastest knockout in the IFL.

CHAPTER FIVE

TOUGH LOVE

"The way you think, the way you behave, the way you eat, can influence your life by 30 to 50 years."
—*Deepak Chopra*

During the years, I have taken note of certain personality types, particularly the one that comes to class, mostly on time and usually with the appropriate gear. Basically, they've shown up, punched in on the old time clock and are there – at least in body.

For some reason, these people aren't quite there in spirit.

I always make it a point to establish a personal relationship with all of my students. I want to know about their job, their family and their pets, in addition to their goals, medical history and personal variants. Because of this, I am able to be a better coach to that person and gain a deeper understanding of their motivation.

All too often, these people show up ready to go, but slowly start to offer less and less during class. They are just going through the motions.

It is no wonder they've maintained the same body shape for the past two years, or gained a few pounds the last few months, or don't have energy like they used to, or "were just so busy today they're going to take it easy."

I believe in hard work, accountability, and positive motivation. I personally work harder when I am happy and have the support of those around me. I constantly try to create the same environment for my students. Unfortunately, this does not work for everybody.

And then it hit me!

Not all people need to be treated with kid gloves; some people need to be hit with a hammer! And, that is what I started doing when nothing else worked. It went something like this:

"What are you doing?! You have legs and arms and healthy organs that allow you to get out of bed every day and walk into my class so you can do WHAT? Waste your time? Waste my time? I don't care if you can't do a single push-up, all I want is for you to try – or leave!"

Well, you get the picture.

Sometimes, we have to tell people what they don't want to hear, because hearing it could potentially save their lives. And sometimes, we need to drop the pretense of our own insecurities and recognize when a friend or loved one is trying to help us, not hurt us.

CHAPTER SIX

CRABS IN THE POT

"All men dream but not equally. Those who dream by night in the dusty recesses of their minds wake in the day to find that it was vanity; but the dreamers of the day are dangerous men, for they may act their dream with open eyes to make it possible."
—T.E. Lawrence

I'm blessed. As a coach, I've mentored the troubled kid, the suit-and-tie professional, the party boy, and the family man, to name a few. My stable of athletes is gorgeous. Thoroughbreds. Work horses.

However, I get the most joy out of helping the every-man and every-woman. When people started asking for *3 Weeks to Shredded* to be mass produced, I shrugged my shoulders and said, "Okay." Not in a million years did I expect to sell as many copies as we have, or receive absolutely tear-jerking testimonials of success from total strangers.

You might be surprised how many of these letters describe them reaching their goals despite the crowds of unsupportive people who surround them. We all face challenges, but it's how we react when faced with these obstacles that make the difference between winning and losing.

Below is part of an actual letter I received. It's from a 54-year-old woman halfway to her goal of losing 40 lbs. At the point I received this letter, she was down 20 lbs. During her weight loss, her sister began bringing a friend to her house. What would you do in this situation?

Mike,

My sister and her friend are here. Her friend likes to cook for us. Last time he was here he made pasta, hot sausage and garlic bread. Tonight, he made breaded steak, garlic bread and potatoes. He tries to bully me into eating with them. It's so hard for me. I say no, and he says, "You cannot starve yourself!" I'M NOT STARVING! I'm losing weight. I'm doing so well. I have to keep my eyes on the prize. It's all very

upsetting to me. I feel like I want to punch him in the face. I don't need to argue with this guy I don't know.
—Shelly

Here's part of what I wrote back:

Shelly,

Just like you have taken control of your life you must now take control of your kitchen. It is YOUR kitchen after all and in MY kitchen, I make the rules. There are no unhealthy ingredients allowed to be brought into my home. If my family and I do feel like we deserve to get some ice cream or enjoy a pizza, we get in the car and make a day of it. My house, just like my body, is my temple.

A major part of every lifestyle change is what I call, "The Crabs in the Pot Syndrome." As a former fisherman, I would notice how crabs would climb on top of each other to get to the top of a holding pot but sure enough, every time one brave little crab got close enough to break free, all of the other crabs would reach up and pull it right back down.

Whether they are trying to pull themselves up with you or simply trying to stop you from enjoying a freedom that they are not yet able to enjoy, does not matter.

We need to recognize these "crabs" in our own life and extract ourselves from their influence. Sometimes it is a coworker, whom we can simply avoid. Other times, it is a family member we cannot avoid, but we can remove their influence over our life choices. In time, you will see that you have become an example to which they will aspire.

Mostly, you must be strong and realize that you are allowed to live your life according to your rules...especially in your own home!

Great work, Shelly! Keep us posted on your progress.
—Mike

I get letters like these all the time:
The coworkers, the friends, the spouse or boyfriend/girlfriend don't understand my goals.
They don't think I need to lose weight.
They're all overweight and so they don't know why I'm doing this.
My boss keeps trying to get me to eat a donut.

ENOUGH!

People, the word is "no." Unfortunately, it sometimes must also be "NO!" People who continually try to force you to stray from your path have been called many things throughout history – all negative in connotation. Think about it.

YOU ARE YOUR OWN BEST CHAMPION!

That's right. YOU! Not your best friend. Not your spouse. Not your child. While everyone around you can cheer you on and be supportive of your endeavors, in actuality the only person you can 100 percent rely on is YOURSELF!

Conversely, you are your own worst enemy. The mind can be a terrible thing. Our thoughts can break us down and create emotional obstacles. More often than not, it is the barriers we erect for ourselves that cause us to fail. Fantastically, our success is also reached by overcoming these false impediments.

GIVE YOURSELF PERMISSION TO KICK ASS

Yes, that's right. Many people put themselves last and only wait to take care of their bodies until it's too late, until heart issues pop up, diabetes sets in, or worse.

Henry David Thoreau said, "Go confidently in the direction of your dreams. Live the life you have imagined." And till this day, I'm blown away by this kid who did just that. Justin B.

Following your dreams and sticking to your goals takes guts. My Grams calls it chutzpah. There are many obstacles along the way in the form of doubts, naysayers and warm, delectable pastries. I know. I've been there and done it many times over. But 23-year-old Justin had been through the emotional ringer and because of that he never lost sight of his goal. He wasn't taken seriously. Girls didn't look at him as a potential boyfriend. He was filled with self-doubt. Then one day, he said ENOUGH! And he flipped the switch to jumpstart his life.

The following is part of his real testimonial that he posted on MyDolceDiet.com – I had never met or heard from Justin before this. He was a complete stranger.

Alright, so I'm new to this site as of today, but I'm certainly not new to Mike Dolce and The Dolce Diet. With his help, I was able to accomplish a dream of mine that I always had, and it was a dream that I never thought could become reality. But thanks to him, and just some hard work, dedication and inspiration, I am sitting here today at a healthy 172 lbs. after weighing in last February 1st at 340 lbs. (in just over a year).

In the beginning, I never thought I'd be able to last on a diet, but after such tremendous reviews, I felt like I owed it to myself, my family, and most importantly my health and body to give it a shot. So that's what I did.

In the first month weight was pouring off of me, which was the spark I needed! Within the first few months my mindset had changed as well. I no longer wanted to cut 40 lbs. or so and then go back to my old self. I wanted to lose so much more weight, and most importantly, continue on this path of a healthy lifestyle.

It felt good to wake up in the morning, see the sun shining, eat a healthy breakfast, hear the birds chirping, do some cardio, hit the gym, and feel refreshed! This was, is, and forever will be the most special and most surreal feeling I could ever feel.

No longer am I "the fat kid," "the nice overweight guy," and all those other things. I feel like I get FULL respect now whether it be at my job, from my family, from girls that would NEVER give me a chance that now suddenly want my number (NO THANKS! I'm still the SAME gentleman, but with a NEW body! If I was NO good for you then, you're NO good for me now! lol)

But seriously, I walk around with confidence and thanks to Mike, I dream bigger things, and I have the confidence that I can, and that I WILL achieve those dreams!

Now that my goal is reached, I'm not taking my foot off the gas pedal. It's now time to maintain this healthy lifestyle, which I will have no problem at all doing. It's more than just enjoyable; it's simply a beautiful, special thing that means the world to me – living life this way. It's unreal.
—Justin B.

After he posted this on the site, Justin received a lot of nice comments. As you could imagine, losing that much weight is a life-changing experience. And while Justin thanks me, I'm more humbled than flattered. Justin is the one who did all the work, not me. I appreciate him taking the time to write about his experience. I absolutely love that he feels right in his own body now. Justin was missing out on the joys life had to offer, and one day he said ENOUGH! and forever changed his life. That's a gutsy move.

CHAPTER SEVEN

DON'T COUNT CALORIES, MAKE CALORIES COUNT

"Nobody creates a fad. It just happens. People love going along with the idea of a beautiful pig. It's like a conspiracy."
—*Jim Henson*

We've all heard the famous Chinese proverb: "Give a man a fish and you feed him for a day. Teach a man to fish and you feed him for a lifetime."

The same principle can be applied to health and wellness. Teach a person how to grocery shop, cook well-balanced recipes, mesh healthy eating habits into their busy lives and make positive choices, and they will be set for life.

Hand them a pre-manufactured frozen TV dinner and – well, you can see where this is going, right?

The diet and exercise industry has the largest amount of fads than any other. Simply stated, any diet that requires the subject to eat a decreased amount of calories for a set period of time will be a diet that, in some capacity, works. Will the person learn how to feed him or herself for the long term? Maybe. Will he or she keep the weight off? Probably not.

The Dolce Diet works because it is not a diet. It is a set of common-sense principles that, when applied, outlines a way of eating for longevity. The results are energy, increased vitality, overall vibrancy and a brighter outlook and yes, when portioned correctly, weight loss.

I don't believe in counting calories. I don't believe in using artificial anything. Why? Because we don't need to count calories if we're eating clean. What is the calorie count of grilled chicken breast, steamed broccoli and a palm-full of quinoa? Who cares?

The only time I notice people counting calories is when they're eating something they shouldn't be.

Your calorie expenditure fluctuates easily from day to day even if your schedule appears to be exactly the same. We must eat based on our actions, not our emotions. A fork in the road does not warrant a spoon in the mouth.

For example, you thought this Monday would be like every other Monday – but you walk in to work to find out those reports are due today, not tomorrow; the boss is breathing down your neck; your computer just exploded, and the copy machine is leaking something gnarly. Oh, and your kid's school nurse called. His temperature is 102.

Now you are burning more calories than usual through accelerated cognitive function and increased physical activity. You go get your kid and take him to the doctor, so you get home two hours later than usual. You now get to the gym late and all the treadmills are taken so instead of a light run you do squats.

All these things add up and it's drastically different compared to Tuesday, when there's no work to be done because you did it all Monday, the kid is healthy and your schedule is back on track, so you get to go home and take a nap before you head to the gym – on time! The difference in calories you've expended on Monday compared with Tuesday is dramatic.

Most people make the mistake of following a general template diet that restricts calories or food groups and shows no regard for energy expenditure. The sample meal plans outlined in this book show you how whole foods consumed often and in great variety is the true secret to *Living Lean*.

Be accountable for what goes into your body.

Be honest with yourself.

CHAPTER EIGHT

GROCERY SHOPPING 101

Go into your kitchen; open your cabinets and pantry. Take everything out and put it on the table. Next, open your refrigerator and do the same thing. Take a good look at what's there. This is what your organs, bones, muscles, dreams and realities are made of. We absorb everything we put into our bodies regardless of its ability to make us healthy or sick, strong or weak.

Below is a handy guide to healthy shopping. Many people eat poorly simply because they shop poorly. Supermarkets are set up like casinos. It is a maze of marketing and strategy, so when you walk into any store, always have a plan.

As soon as you enter most markets, you will see the produce section, which houses the fruits and vegetables. Always start your shopping here and only pick up items from your list. I have made one for you to use as a reference.

GROCERY LIST

Fruit	Green Vegetables	Colored Vegetables
Strawberries	Baby spinach	Tomatoes
Blueberries	Green peppers	Red peppers
Apples	Asparagus	Onions
Oranges	Broccoli	Beets
Mangos	Kale	Carrots
Avocados	Zucchini	Corn
Bananas	Brussels sprouts	Sweet potatoes

Grains	Nuts	Legume
Oat bran	Walnuts	Garbanzo beans
Quinoa	Cashews	Black beans
Brown rice	Pistachios	Kidney beans
Pasta	Almond butter	Pinto beans
Ezekial low-sodium	Peanut butter	Red beans
bread	Hazelnuts	Fava beans
Buckwheat	Pecans	Lima beans
Amaranth		

Fats	Dairy/Non-Dairy	Animal Protein
Flax seeds	**Alternative**	Eggs
Chia seeds	Almond milk	Wild red salmon
Peanut oil	Coconut milk	Tuna
Grapeseed oil	Feta cheese	Chicken breast
Coconut oil	Havarti cheese	Ground turkey
Extra virgin olive oil	Mozzarella cheese	
Hemp oil	Rice cheddar cheese	
	Almond cheese	

These items should always be on hand: Purified water, green tea, basil, oregano, fresh garlic, thyme, paprika, sea salt, pepper, rosemary, cayenne, turmeric, cumin, and cinnamon.

BUYER BEWARE

While shopping, remember that product labels are designed to attract you. They are a sales tactic. For instance, many people confuse nonfat vs. fat products.

Nonfat does not necessarily mean less calories or "better for you." Often nonfat foods have more sugar in them than their regular-fat counterparts. And certain so-called "sugar-free" foods are often sweetened with suspicious chemicals. (Google *danger+splenda* and see what pops up.)

You must read the ingredients.

THE NUTRITION FACTS LABEL

Most people glance at a product and only look at the calories. Some go a little bit further and compare the fat, carbohydrate and protein content.

Many don't even consider the fiber content, but the key concern really should be with the fine print: The ingredients. That is where you actually find out what you're eating.

Protein, carbohydrate and fat quality will differ drastically depending on what the item is made of. You only find this through the ingredients, which are listed in order of their quantity in the product. That means the first ingredient on the list makes up the largest amount of the product and so on.

CHAPTER NINE

STRUCTURING A MEAL PLAN

The Four Types of Nutritional Motivation

In my experience, the four most common meal plans are focused on:

1. Athletes
2. Health & Wellness
3. Gluten-Free
4. Vegan

Each of us has a specific goal in mind and those goals will often change with time. Some goals are strictly based upon performance or body composition while others may be focused on general health or even ecology. Each of these forms a basic motivation to follow a specific meal plan, or nutritional lifestyle.

The goal of *Living Lean* is to outline a simple structure in which each of the four primary lifestyles can actually converge and follow the same exact meal plan, with a few easy exchanges.

For example, my family and I have varied personal goals and often follow different nutritional lifestyles, yet we can eat virtually the same meal with a few simple alterations.

I believe in a holistic approach to health and it is very important to embrace the positive social and emotional impact of sitting with your family or friends while you eat. This builds a very strong support system regardless of your goal, and makes the time spent preparing your meals much more rewarding.

This concept is very important.

I have the experience of working closely with many elite athletes who support their families as a result of their athletic performance, yet have a hard time following a proper meal plan simply because it is too difficult to feed the kids one meal, mom a different meal and the athlete another. More often than not, the athlete would eat closer to what the kids were eating, sacrificing his own goals.

Maybe this is you too?

All of the meals outlined in *Living Lean* can and should be enjoyed by the entire family with very minor additions or subtractions to fit each member's goal.

For example, a few weeks ago, while I was in a Health & Wellness stage following a Gluten-Free nutritional lifestyle, my wife was in an Athletic stage and had planned a pasta meal to fuel her training for an upcoming race. My sister was coming to dinner with her 3-year-old son, both of whom are Vegan and Gluten-modified. This may present a dilemma to some hosts who might not know what to make to keep everyone happy. But, for those of us following the principles of *Living Lean*, you will be fine!

My Power Pasta Sauce is completely organic, gluten-free and vegan. That means ANYbody can eat it and still stay within their own nutritional lifestyle.

My wife and I had a blast cooking the sauce, sipping a glass of red wine and sharing quality time in the kitchen while everyone else kept popping over to the stove, saying, "Wow, that smells great!"

The only changes we made to our menu were to add a pot of quinoa, a gluten-free option, in addition to a pot of whole wheat pasta. Both are vegan approved.

We also offered slices of fresh mozzarella, grated parmesan cheese, a vibrant green spinach salad, toasted brown rice bread and sprouted grain bread with a touch of extra virgin olive oil and balsamic vinegar for dipping.

Everybody loved the meal, ate 100 percent within their nutritional lifestyle...and there wasn't a single scrap of food left over! Again, the purpose of this book is to show you how easy it is to LIVE LEAN!

Below is a sample meal plan that can be used by athlete and obese alike. Feel free to personalize this plan with different recipes to suit your lifestyle. Pay close attention to the Health, Vegan, and Gluten-Free options. All recipes are listed in the next chapter.

A= Athlete
H=Health-Minded
G=Gluten-Free
V=Vegan (no animal products)

BREAKFAST 6:30 am

16 oz. water & "The Breakfast Bowl" (A, H, G, V)

*Coffee or tea can be drunk AFTER breakfast has been eaten.

SNACK 10:00 am

1 apple & 2 Tbsp. almond butter (A, H, G, V)

LUNCH 1:00 pm

16 oz. water & 1 cup green tea

"Egg Scramble"

3 whole eggs (A, H, G)

or 3 egg whites (A, H, G)

or ½ cup quinoa (A, H, G, V)

MID-DAY SNACK 4:00 pm

(A, H, G, V)

2 slices UDI's gluten-free bread (toasted)

1 Tbsp. almond butter

1 Tbsp. agave

7:00 pm		
Monday & Thursday	Tuesday & Friday	Wednesday & Saturday
Dinner:	**Dinner:**	**Dinner:**
16 oz. water	16 oz. water	16 oz. water
(A, H, G)	(A, H, G, V)	(A, H, G)
Chicken Dinner	**Chick Pea Salad**	**Salmon Dinner**
6 oz. chicken breast	6 oz. chick peas	8 oz. fresh salmon
2 cups asparagus	2 cups baby spinach	2 cups broccoli
1 cup/ear of corn	1 cup kale	1 cup carrots
½ cup quinoa	½ cucumber	½ cup cooked
	¼ chopped onion	brown rice
	½ tomato	
	½ chopped walnuts	
	6 sliced strawberries	
	*4 oz. feta cheese	
	crumbles	
	3 Tbsp. hemp oil	
	3 Tbsp. balsamic vinegar	
	*(optional – not Vegan)	

10:00 pm		
Monday & Thursday	Tuesday & Friday	Wednesday & Saturday
Dessert:	**Dessert:**	**Dessert:**
(A, H, G)	(A, H, V)	(A, H, G, V)
1 cup chamomile tea	1 cup chamomile tea	1 cup chamomile tea
½ cup plain yogurt	1 cup Kashi Autumn	2 slices Udi's toast
1 cup blueberries	Wheat	1 Tbsp. agave
1 Tbsp. agave	½ banana	1 Tbsp. almond butter
	Almond milk	

CHAPTER TEN

RECIPES FROM INSIDE MMA'S ELITE FIGHT CAMPS

All of the ingredients in these recipes are optional. By now, you have learned the principles of *Living Lean*. Feel free to be creative! Experiment! Make each recipe your own. Just use good nutritional judgment when doing so.

Here are some tips to remember:

- Unless otherwise noted, all ingredients are to be as close to their natural state as possible. That means they should be fresh, organic, free-range, local, non-processed and not genetically modified.
- For cooking, use coconut, grapeseed, and/or peanut oil. They remain stable at medium to high heats.
- Extra virgin olive oil is not a cooking oil and should never be served above room temperature.
- A dash is about 1/8 of a teaspoon.
- A pinch is about half of a dash.

NUTRITIONAL MOTIVATION KEY

A= Athlete

H=Health-Minded

G=Gluten-Free

V=Vegan (no animal products)

BREAKFAST

Certainly the most important meal of the day is breakfast. If we could only eat a well-balanced breakfast, as opposed to a well-balanced dinner each day, the breakfast eaters would be much healthier, capable individuals.

It surprises me when a modern adult admits to regularly missing breakfast. As the first meal of the day, it must be the first thing you do. There may be places to go and things to do afterward, but you must start with breakfast.

Most people begin their day with coffees, teas and juices before addressing the most basic human need: WATER. If you are thirsty, you are dehydrated. The first thing you should do every morning is sip room-temperature, filtered water. This will clean your digestive tract, begin revitalizing your cells and fire up your metabolism.

Now, prepare your ingredients, turn on the teapot and take a minute to enjoy the beginning of a wonderful day!

BREAKFAST BOWL

(A, H, G ,V)

½ cup oat bran or buckwheat (G)

1 cup blueberries

½ cup strawberries

¼ cup raisins

½ sliced banana

1 Tbsp. all-natural peanut or almond butter

1 Tbsp. ground flax seeds

1 pinch cinnamon

1 cup water

- In a medium saucepan bring 1 cup water to boil.
- Reduce flame and mix in berries and oat bran, stirring often until desired consistency is reached.
- Mix in flax seeds, raisins and cinnamon.
- Pour into bowl and add peanut butter or almond butter and top with banana.
- Add in a dash of almond milk or water to thin out oat bran if desired.

PITBULL PANCAKES

(A, H, G, V)

1 cup Pamela's Baking & Pancake Mix

1 large egg *or egg alternative* (V)*

3/4 cup water

1 Tbsp. coconut oil

- Follow the pancake directions on the back of the Pamela's mix.
- Use coconut oil for the mix *and* to cook the pancakes.
- Serve with **Fresh Berry Syrup**.

NOTE: Add more water to batter for thinner pancakes. Less water for thicker pancakes.

EASY EGG ALTERNATIVE (I EGG)

1 Tbsp. ground flax seeds

3 Tbsp. water

- Stir together until thick and gelatinous

EAST COAST BREAKFAST TOAST

(A, H, G, V)

1 egg (or egg alternative)

¼ cup almond milk

2 slices bread

Coconut oil (as needed)

1 dash cinnamon

- Coat pan with coconut oil and place over low heat.
- In bowl, beat eggs and milk together with fork.
- Dip bread into egg mixture and soak through.
- Put bread slices in pan and heat until lightly browned.
- Be sure to flip them over to cook both sides.
- Repeat until all bread slices have been browned.
- Top each bread slice with cinnamon, fresh fruit or serve with **Fresh Berry Syrup**.
- If cooking for more than one person, just double the recipe as you see fit.

FRESH BERRY SYRUP

(A, H, G, V)

4 oz. water

1 cup strawberries

1 cup blueberries

1 Tbsp. agave *(optional)*

- Add water and fruit to small sauce pan.
- Cover and turn to low-medium heat.
- When fruit softens, reduce heat and mash with spatula.
- Add agave, stir and serve.

OATS & BERRIES SMOOTHIE

(A, H, G, V)

1 cup blueberries

1 cup strawberries

1 orange

1 banana

½ cup uncooked oat bran *or buckwheat (G)*

½ cup almond milk

1 Tsp. honey

10 ice cubes

- Combine in blender and blend until creamy.

LUNCH

Lunch is best kept simple. We all get very busy, especially in the middle of the day, which is why we should plan our lunches the night before. The recipes that follow are very easy to make and are designed to be portable, while being delicious. As a rule, bring your lunch with you. You cannot rely on having the time to find a proper meal in the middle of a hectic day.

Sometimes, I'll grab a container filled with Salmon Salad, a loaf of Ezekial bread, a few apples, and throw everything in my cooler. Even if I plan on being home for lunch, I may get diverted or stuck in traffic, but I'm prepared.

SALMON SALAD

(A, H, G)

1 can wild-caught Alaskan Sockeye

½ stalk celery, chopped

¼ cup red or sweet onion, chopped

2 Tsp. spicy brown mustard or horseradish

2 Tbsp. dill pickle relish (unsweetened)

1/4 Tsp. black pepper

7 pitted black olives, chopped *(optional)*

½ avocado

Brown rice wrap or bread

- Put salmon in a large mixing bowl and mash in celery, onion, mustard, relish, olives, pepper and avocado.
- Mix thoroughly, mashing avocado into the mixture.
- Transfer mixture to brown rice wrap or bread. Enjoy!

CHICK PEA SALAD

(A, H, G, V)

6 oz. chick peas (garbanzo beans)

1 handful baby spinach

1 handful kale

½ cucumber, sliced

¼ chopped onion

½ tomato, chopped - or 6 cherry tomatoes

½ cup chopped walnuts

6 sliced strawberries

4 oz. feta cheese crumbles *(optional)*

3 Tbsp. extra virgin olive oil

3 Tbsp. balsamic vinegar

- Combine all ingredients in bowl and drizzle with olive oil and balsamic vinegar.

EGG SALAD

(A, H, G)

4 whole hard boiled eggs, peeled and chopped

¼ onion, chopped

1 dash sea salt

1 dash black pepper

½ avocado

Bread or wrap

- Combine eggs, onion, salt and pepper in mixing bowl.
- Scoop out half an avocado and add to mixture.
- Mash well.
- Serve on whole wheat or gluten-free bread, in wrap or over salad.

TUNA SALAD

(A, H, G)

1 can tuna in water

¼ onion, chopped

½ celery stalk, chopped

½ avocado

1-2 Tbsp. brown spicy mustard

1 Tbsp. sweet pickle relish

1 hard-boiled egg

- Mix all ingredients together and put on whole wheat or gluten-free bread, in wrap or enjoy over green salad.

SUPAFLY CHICKEN SALAD

(A, H, G)

8 oz. chicken breast, cut into bite-sized pieces

½ celery stalk, chopped

1 cup grapes, halved

1 cup chick peas

1 avocado, peeled and pitted

1 Tsp. lemon juice

Sea salt and pepper, to taste

- Lightly coat pan with grapeseed oil and cook chicken over low-medium heat.
- Combine rest of ingredients in large bowl and mix well, mashing avocado into mixture.
- Once chicken is cooked, let cool and then add to rest of ingredients in bowl and mix well.
- Chill until serving.
- This salad can be served a number of ways: On a bed of lettuce, on whole grain bread or in a gluten-free wrap.

OMELET

(A, H, G)

3 whole eggs

¼ diced red pepper

¼ diced onion

¼ cup almond milk

1 cup mushrooms, sliced

1 handful spinach leaves

1 dash sea salt

1 slice Havarti cheese *(optional)*

1/3 avocado, smeared on toast

2 slices toasted bread

- Lightly coat 2 medium sauté pans with grapeseed oil and put on low heat.
- Dice peppers, onions and mushrooms. Add to pan #1. Sauté for about 2 minutes and add mushrooms.
- Whip eggs and milk in medium mixing bowl.
- Once the vegetables begin to soften, add spinach leaves to pan #1.
- Once spinach has begun to wilt, remove pan #1 from heat.
- Evenly pour eggs into pan #2 so they coat the bottom of the pan and cover. (Do not stir.)
- Once hard, flip the omelet over and immediately add contents of pan #1 and cheese slice to half of the omelet. Fold the empty omelet half over on top and serve with toast smeared with avocado.

EGG SCRAMBLE

(A, H, G)

3 whole eggs

¼ diced red pepper

¼ diced onion

1 cup mushrooms, sliced

1 handful spinach leaves

1 dash sea salt

1 slice white cheese *(optional)*

1/3 avocado, smeared on toast

2 slices toasted bread

- Lightly coat medium sauté pan with grapeseed oil and put on low heat.
- Dice peppers and onions and add to pan. Sauté about 2 minutes, then add mushrooms.
- Whip eggs in medium mixing bowl.
- Once the peppers, onions and mushrooms soften, add spinach leaves.
- Once spinach begins to wilt, evenly pour eggs into pan.
- Lightly stir into a scramble.
- Once desired consistency is reached, turn off stovetop, mix in cheese and serve with toast smeared with avocado.

STRAWBERRY SALAD

(A, H, G, V)

2 handfuls baby spinach

10 fresh strawberries, sliced

½ avocado, cut into bite-sized chunks

1 cup walnuts

Arrange spinach, avocado, walnuts and strawberries in bowl.

Dressing: Light drizzle of extra virgin olive oil and balsamic vinegar

PASTA SALAD WITH VEGGIES

(A, H, G, V)

2 cups rotini pasta or gluten-free pasta, cooked according to package instructions and drained

1 cup chopped broccoli, steamed

1 cup chick peas

1/3 cup cubed or shredded mozzarella cheese *(optional)*

1 clove garlic, minced

½ tomato, diced

Dressing: Light drizzle of extra virgin olive oil and balsamic vinegar

- In a bowl, mix all ingredients together. Cool in refrigerator until ready to serve. To serve, add dressing and cheese.

SIMPLE SPINACH SALAD

(A, H, G, V)

This is a great weight-cutting meal when you need to be light but want to keep your energy high.

1 handful fresh spinach leaves

1 handful colored vegetable, chopped

1 handful fruit, chopped

Dressing: Light drizzle of hemp oil and apple cider vinegar

- Mix all ingredients in bowl and top with dressing.

WALDORF SALAD

(A, H, G)

½ cup chopped walnuts

½ cup plain yogurt

2 Tbsp. avocado

2 Tbsp. parsley, minced

1 Tsp. honey

Freshly ground black pepper to taste

2 large apples, chopped into ½ inch pieces

2 celery stalks, chopped

¼ cup raisins

½ lemon, juiced

1 head Romaine lettuce, shredded into bite-sized pieces

- Mix yogurt, avocado, parsley, honey and pepper in a bowl.
- Add the apples, celery and raisins and sprinkle with the lemon juice; toss with yogurt mixture.
- Wait to add walnuts and lettuce until you're ready to eat the salad.
- Chill before serving.

DRESSINGS

OIL & VINEGAR DRESSING

Extra virgin olive oil, add to taste
Balsamic vinegar, add to taste

NATURE'S DRESSING

Hemp oil, add to taste
Apple cider vinegar, add to taste

GRAPESEED PESTO

1 ½ cups fresh basil leaves
½ cup grapeseed oil

- Grind basil to a fine paste with mortar and pestle* and put in small bowl.
- Add grapeseed oil and stir.

You can also use a blender or food processor.

STRAWBERRY VINAIGRETTE

½ cup extra virgin olive oil
½ pint fresh strawberries, halved
2 Tbsp. balsamic vinegar
½ Tsp. sea salt
¼ Tsp. black pepper

- Blend all ingredients until smooth. Serve over salad.

DINNER

The dinner table of many hardworking, well-intentioned families has been taken over by grab-n-go burgers and pizza delivery. Stop this now! The following recipes are simple, nutritious, cost effective and easily modified to your taste.

CHICKEN & ASPARAGUS STIR FRY

(A, H, G)

2 chicken breasts cut into bite-sized pieces

1 bunch thin asparagus (about 20 stalks)

2 cloves garlic, chopped

1 medium shallot, minced

2 Tbsp. low-sodium soy sauce or teriyaki sauce

- Cut off thick ends of asparagus; wash what remains and cut into bite-sized pieces.
- Steam for about 7-10 minutes, or until bright green, and then set aside.
- In a large pan, sauté shallot and garlic in peanut oil for about 2 minutes.
- Add chicken and continue to sauté about 6 minutes or until pink disappears.
- Pour into heat-safe serving bowl and mix in asparagus.
- Add 2 Tbsp. low-sodium soy sauce or teriyaki sauce and serve.

SAUTÉED GARLIC & MUSHROOM STRING BEANS

(A, H, G, V)

2 lbs. fresh (or frozen) organic green beans

9 large shiitake mushrooms (fresh, not dried)

4-5 medium cloves of garlic, minced

- Wash beans, cut off ends, and snap them in half.
- Steam the green beans until tender. Drain and set aside.
- Coat large pan with grapeseed oil and place on low-medium heat.
- Add garlic and mushrooms and cook for 3 minutes, stirring occasionally.
- Mix in the green beans and sauté for 6-8 minutes, until beans are browned.
- Serve with quinoa, fish or chicken.

TURKEY BURGERS

(A, H, G)

½ lb. lean turkey

¼ cup oat bran *or buckwheat (G)*

1 whole egg

2 cloves garlic, chopped

1 Tsp. Worcestershire or teriyaki sauce

1 dash each of sea salt, pepper and oregano

Optional toppings

Romaine lettuce

Sliced tomato

Dill pickle

Avocado

Cheese

Ketchup

Mustard

- Lightly coat pan with grapeseed oil and set on low-medium heat.
- In a large bowl, combine everything except toppings and mix well.
- Shape into 4 to 5 palm-sized patties.
- Place patties in pan and flatten with spatula.
- Grill, covered, over indirect medium heat for 4-6 minutes on each side or until meat is no longer pink inside.
- Serve on bread or wrapped in lettuce with optional toppings.

FIGHTER FAJITAS

(A, H, G, V)

1 lb. skinless, boneless chicken breasts

Or 16 oz. black beans (V)

1 Tsp. chili powder

½ Tsp. sea salt

½ Tsp. ground cumin

½ Tsp. freshly ground black pepper

8-12 whole wheat or gluten-free tortillas

For toppings:

1 avocado, mashed in bowl with 1 Tbsp. lemon juice. Set aside.

1 chopped tomato

¼ head of lettuce, chopped

Shredded cheddar cheese *(optional)*

- Preheat oven to 350 degrees F.
- Coat pan in grapeseed oil and set on low-medium heat.
- Combine chili powder, sea salt, cumin and black pepper in a small bowl.
- Chop raw chicken in bite-sized pieces and sprinkle with spices.
- Place chicken in pan and cook 10 minutes, stirring often, until done.
- Heat tortillas on cookie sheet in oven for 2 minutes and remove.
- Divide chicken evenly among tortillas; top each tortilla with a sprinkle of lettuce, tomato, avocado and cheese.

HONEY GLAZED SALMON

(A, H, G)

8 oz. wild-caught salmon

Sea salt

Honey

- Coat small pan with grapeseed oil and put on low-medium heat
- Rub salmon with grapeseed oil and sprinkle with sea salt.
- Cook 3-5 minutes on each side, depending on thickness.
- Salmon should be cooked evenly through the center.
- Plate and drizzle with honey.

POWER PASTA SAUCE

(A, H, G, V)

This sauce can be made several ways and can be mixed with everything or nothing. This sauce makes a great dip for bread, serve it over pasta or chicken, or mix with rice or quinoa for a hearty meal.

16 oz. pasta (whole wheat, durum, brown rice, quinoa or gluten-free pasta noodles)

4 - 16 oz. cans of diced tomatoes or 12-14 whole tomatoes, steamed, peeled and crushed

1 red pepper, chopped

1 green pepper, chopped

1 medium sweet onion, chopped

10-12 cloves garlic, diced

1 pinch each of basil, oregano and sea salt

16 oz. organic ground turkey *(optional – not vegan)*

Extra virgin olive oil

Grapeseed oil

- Pour diced tomatoes in large pot and heat over low-medium flame.
- Add basil, oregano and sea salt before covering to simmer.
- Sauté garlic, onion and peppers in grapeseed oil over low-medium heat.
- In another pan at low-medium heat, begin to brown the turkey in grapeseed oil.
- In another large pot, bring 6-8 cups water to boil.
- Once vegetables have softened to your taste, add to sauce.
- When turkey has thoroughly cooked, add to sauce, cover and simmer another 10 minutes before removing from heat.
- Add pasta noodles to boiling water and cook for 8-12 minutes.
- Stir in 2 Tbsp. extra virgin olive oil.
- When noodles are done, add separately to plates and cover with sauce.

GARLIC PORTABELLA CHICKEN WITH ASPARAGUS & SPINACH

(A, H, G, V)

½ chicken breast, cut into bite-sized pieces

(Vegan: eliminate chicken and use whole portabella mushroom top)

1/3 portabella mushroom, chopped

1 handful baby spinach

1 Tbsp. garlic, minced

Half bunch asparagus (6-8 stalks), steamed

1 dash each of sea salt, oregano and pepper

- Coat medium pan with grapeseed oil and put on low-medium heat.
- Add portabella mushroom and garlic to pan.
- Once mushrooms brown, add handful of spinach leaves and sauté until spinach shrinks into mushroom mixture.
- Add asparagus.
- In separate pan, sprinkle chicken with spices and sauté in grapeseed oil.
- Once cooked, add chicken to mushroom pan. Lightly stir mixture.
- Let cook together for 5 minutes, then plate.

SKINNY SUMO STIR FRY

(A, H, G ,V)

1 chicken breast, cut into bite-sized pieces

(Vegan: instead of chicken, serve over quinoa)

2 cups broccoli, chopped

1 cup mushrooms, chopped

1 Tbsp. low-sodium soy sauce

4 green onions, chopped

1 handful bean sprouts

- Coat small pan with peanut oil and cook chicken until no longer pink inside.
- Steam broccoli in separate pan until tender.
- In another pan, sauté mushrooms in peanut oil until browned.
- Combine chicken, mushrooms and broccoli in bowl.
- Top with onions, sprouts and low-sodium soy sauce.

BAKED CHICKEN DINNER

(A, H, G)

1 chicken breast, sliced horizontally

1 dash sea salt

1 dash pepper

- Preheat oven to 350 degrees F.
- Rub chicken with grapeseed oil and sprinkle with sea salt and pepper. Place in baking dish and cook for 20 minutes or until no longer pink inside.

SPINACH PASTA

(A, H, G, V)

16 oz. whole-wheat or brown rice noodles, or 1 cup quinoa

1 handful fresh baby spinach

1 cup basil leaves, tightly packed

3 cloves garlic, minced

1 Tbsp. grapeseed oil

1/3 cup almond milk

½ cup mozzarella cheese, shredded *(optional – not vegan)*

Sea salt and pepper to taste

- Cook pasta according to package directions.
- Chop spinach and basil in blender or food processor. If you don't have a chopping appliance, just shred by hand.
- In a large saucepan, sauté garlic in grapeseed oil.
- Add milk and spinach mixture to saucepan. Bring to a boil, then reduce heat to a simmer. Stir occasionally until sauce slightly thickens and remove from heat.
- Drain water and add noodles to spinach mixture in saucepan. Add cheese, sea salt and pepper. Serve immediately.

CHAMPION CHILI

(A, H, G, V)

½ lb. ground organic turkey *or 1 can chick peas (V)*

2 cans diced tomatoes or 6-7 freshly chopped tomatoes

1 can kidney beans

1 red pepper, chopped

1 green pepper, chopped

1 sweet onion, chopped

4 cloves garlic, chopped

Sea salt, to taste

Chili powder, to taste

- 1 cup shredded rice cheddar cheese *(optional)*
- Put tomatoes and beans in large pot and place on low heat.
- Brown meat in separate pan and add to tomato pot.
- In another pan, sauté peppers, onions and garlic in grapeseed oil. Once tender, add to tomato pot.
- Add sea salt and chili powder to taste.
- Sprinkle with cheese and serve.

COD OR TILAPIA

(A, H, G)

1 cod or tilapia filet

1 dash each of sea salt, rosemary and pepper

½ lemon, juiced

- Heat oven to 350 degrees F.
- Rub fish with grapeseed oil and spices.
- Bake in casserole dish for 15 minutes.
- Squeeze fresh lemon juice over filet and serve.

THORO-BREADED FRIED CHICKEN

(A, H, G)

1 chicken breast, sliced horizontally

1 cup oat bran *or buckwheat (G)*

1 egg

1/3 cup almond milk

1 Tbsp. ground flax seeds

- Mix 1 egg and 1/3 cup milk in small bowl.
- Combine oat bran and flax seeds in separate bowl.
- Coat pan with coconut oil and heat over low-medium flame.
- Dip chicken in egg/milk mixture, and then roll chicken in oat bran/ flax seeds mixture to coat.
- Immediately place in pan. Cook 3-4 minutes on each side.

PINEAPPLE CHICKEN "FRIED" QUINOA

(A, H, G, V)

1 cup uncooked quinoa

1 organic chicken breast, cut into bite-sized pieces

(Vegan: use tofu, extra firm, cubed)

1 cup crushed pineapple

2 eggs, beaten

¾ cup mushrooms, chopped

3 Tbsp. low-sodium soy sauce

3 green onions, thinly sliced

1 cup carrots, diced

- Add 1 cup quinoa and 2 cups water to large saucepan.
- Bring to boil, reduce heat and cover for 15 minutes.
- Coat small pan with coconut oil and cook chicken.
- Coat another small pan with coconut oil and cook eggs without stirring.
- Once solid, put eggs on cutting surface and chop.
- Using egg pan, sauté mushrooms, green onions and carrots until tender.
- Stir in quinoa, pineapple and egg pieces.
- Add chicken to vegetable mixture.
- Add soy sauce and stir. Serve hot.

SNACKS

YOGURT, FRUIT & HONEY BOWL

(A, H, G)

1 cup Greek yogurt or plain yogurt (not vanilla)

1 cup fresh berries

1 Tbsp. honey

- Combine in bowl and enjoy!

TOAST

(A, H, G, V)

- Spread Justin's Chocolate Hazelnut Butter, peanut butter, honey or bananas on your favorite toasted bread.

CLASSIC CEREAL

(A, H, V)

Kashi Autumn Wheat

Pair with almond milk and add dash of cinnamon

Fresh fruit *(optional)*

FRUIT & NUTS

(A, H, G, V)

- Fruit paired with a handful of nuts is an excellent energy boosting snack.
- Check the shopping list in Chapter Eight for ideas.

THE AVOCADO

(A, H, G, V)

- Cut the avocado in half, take out the pit and spoon it out like pudding.
- Pair with an orange or two for a great snack.

GREEN SCHMEAR

(A, H, G, V)

- Smear avocado on bread slice and enjoy.

SIMPLE GUACAMOLE DIP

(A, H, G, V)

2 large, ripe avocados, scooped out

¼ tomato, chopped

2-3 Tbsp. lime juice, to taste

1/3 cup onion, chopped

½ Tsp. chili powder, to taste

½ Tsp. sea salt

Chopped jalapenos *(optional)*

- Combine all ingredients in mixing bowl and mash with fork to desired consistency.

JUICING

As a rule, all fruit and vegetables can be juiced together. That is part of the fun. Storing the leftovers in glass containers goes a long way toward preserving its flavor. Fresh juice has a shelf life of less than a day. Kind of makes you wonder what's in the store-bought stuff. Here are two of my favorite juicing recipes.

BAPPLE JUICE

1 beet with leaves

4 apples

2 sticks celery *(optional)*

2 Tbsp. chia seeds

- Juice beets, apples and celery together and pour into glass.
- Stir in chia seeds and enjoy!

THE KITCHEN SINK

1 whole beet with leaves

4 apples

2 oranges, peeled

1 lemon, peeled

1 cup strawberries

1 handful spinach

4 carrots

3 stalks celery

1 tomato

2 Tbsp. hemp oil

1 golf-ball sized hunk of ginger root

- Juice together and enjoy!

CHAPTER ELEVEN

WORKOUT PRINCIPLES

Let's keep this super simple. In the gym, be efficient. Walk in, put down your gear and get to work. Always begin with a warm-up. This can be as simple as a few minutes of calisthenics or a couple miles on the treadmill. Get your heart rate up and make sure you're sweating before the first exercise.

SETS & REPS

You may need to adjust the sample workouts in this book according to your training experience and goals. Start with your body weight or light weights and adjust from there.

- To gain **strength**, keep the reps at 5-8.
- To gain **muscle**, keep the reps at 8-12.
- To gain **endurance**, keep the reps between 12 and 100.

VOLUME & INTENSITY

Volume is the amount of hours, reps or pounds you total during a given training cycle. Intensity is the level of energy you put into your volume.

If you train very intensely, you must keep your volume at a minimum in order to achieve results. If you train with less intensity, your volume must be higher. If you train with little intensity and little volume, you will achieve little results. If you train at high intensity with high volume, something will break – your body or your spirit.

REST INTERVALS

I prefer to look at rest intervals in terms of deep breathing. Whether it is 15 seconds during a superset or 1 minute between rounds of a championship fight, the goal of rest is to reduce your heart rate through controlled breathing. This allows your body to recover naturally and settles the mind.

FORM

All form must always be perfect. I define perfect as your personal best. I've been strength training for over 20 years, and I still strive to perfect my form.

Adherence to proper form increases the efficiency of the exercise. Poor form often results in injury, strength plateaus and muscular imbalances.

GOAL SETTING

This is the most important factor in any success. Your goals for exercise must be specific *and* general.

- A general goal might be: *I want to lose weight.*
- A specific goal might be: *I will lose 40 lbs. by Christmas.*
- We further break that down to the method by which you will achieve your goal: *I will perform three strength sessions this week as well as two cardiovascular sessions.* Now get specific: *I will perform 20 squats on Monday, 25 on Wednesday, and 30 on Friday.* Or *I will run the same distance during my cardio sessions, but each time finish just a little faster.*

If you do not set a goal walking into a workout, you are simply going through the motions and far reducing your chance of success.

CHAPTER TWELVE

STRENGTH TRAINING WORKOUTS

This chapter offers sample training routines that can be immediately implemented into your own lifestyle. It doesn't matter if you're a professional athlete or stay-at-home mom, there is something in here for you.

QUICK-START WORKOUTS

Not everybody's fighting for the world title, so I don't expect you to train like a professional athlete. The following workouts are designed for everybody.

QUICK-START WORKOUT - CHEST

This is for the suit-and-tie guy just looking to fill out his jacket. You have three days – if you're lucky – to get to the gym each week. This is the workout for you.

WARM-UP

- 3 sets x 25 jumping jacks

BARBELL BENCH PRESS

- 3 sets x 50 reps with an empty bar

INCLINE DUMBBELL PRESS

- 5 sets x 8-12 reps

TWO-ARM BENT-OVER DUMBBELL ROWS

- 3 sets x 8-12 reps (each side)

DUMBBELL SIDE LATERALS

- 2 sets x 15 reps

PUSH-UPS

- 1 set to total failure
- You can also finish with a few sets of biceps curls, sit-ups, or a few minutes on the treadmill.

QUICK-START WORKOUT - ABS

This area calls both men and women alike. If your goal is a slimmer, stronger waistline, this is the workout for you.

Pick five exercises and perform 1 set of 50 reps each (or make that the goal). Today you may only be able to do 1 set of 10 reps of each exercise. Tomorrow, do 11 reps. The next day, do 12. Once you have completed the entire cycle of 5 sets of 50 reps, it's time to add a new cycle.

The goal should be three cycles of five exercises for 50 reps each. When you can do that, your waistline will be the envy of all.

LYING TOE TOUCH

LEG RAISE DOUBLE

X-PATTERN TOE TOUCH

ALTERNATE STRAIGHT LEG CRUNCH

BOSU BALL SUPERMAN ALTERNATE SIDE RAISE

QUICK-START WORKOUT - LEGS

This is a fantastic workout for those looking to tighten the glutes and give definition to calves and thighs.

WARM-UP

- 15-minute walk on treadmill at low incline

FORWARD DUMBBELL LUNGE

- 3 sets x 15 reps (each leg)

BACKWARD DUMBBELL LUNGE

- 3 sets x 15 reps (each leg)

SINGLE LEG DUMBBELL DEADLIFT

- 3 sets x 15 reps (each leg)

POWER SQUAT

- 3 sets x 15 reps

COOL-DOWN

- 15-minute walk on treadmill

FULL BODY FUNCTIONAL WORKOUT

This is the best all-around workout for any one of us to strengthen and shape the entire body while building stamina and flexibility. Take your time here and simply start with just your body weight for as many reps as you can comfortably perform. Initially, some of us may benefit greatly from just one set of 10 reps in each exercise. In time, your reps will go up and you will embrace the challenge of adding more weight.

X-PATTERN TOE TOUCH

3 sets x 15 reps each side

- 30 seconds rest between each set.
- 60 seconds rest between each exercise.

POWER SQUAT

1 set x 25 reps with 25 lb. dumbbells

- 60 seconds rest before next exercise.

TWO-ARM BENT-OVER DUMBBELL ROWS

5 sets x 25 reps with 25 lb. dumbbells

- 30 seconds rest between each set.
- 60 seconds rest between each exercise.

POWER SQUAT

1 set x 25 reps with 25 lb. dumbbells

- 60 seconds rest before next exercise.

CHAIN PUSH-UP

5 sets x 10 reps with 1 chain

- 30 seconds rest between each set.
- 60 seconds rest between each exercise.

POWER SQUAT

1 set x 25 reps with 25 lb. dumbbells

- 60 seconds rest before next exercise.

ELBOW-TO-KNEE BACK EXTENSION

3 sets x 15 reps each side

- 30 seconds rest between each set.
- 60 seconds rest between each exercise.

POWER SQUAT

1 set x 25 reps with 25 lb. dumbbells

TANK TOP WORKOUT #1

This workout is great for ladies looking to tighten and tone or elite athletes looking to maximize upper body endurance. Sets and reps for beginners should be reduced until a mastery of form is achieved.

BOSU BALL PUSH-UP

5 sets x 15 reps

- 30 seconds rest between each set.
- 60 seconds rest between each exercise.

BARBELL BENCH PRESS

1 set x 100 reps with empty bar

- 30 seconds rest.

5 sets x 50 reps with 10 lbs. added to each side of the bar

- 30 seconds rest between each set.
- 60 seconds rest between each exercise.

BARBELL UPRIGHT ROW

3 sets x 20 reps with 5 lbs. on each side of the barbell

- 30 seconds rest between each set.
- 60 seconds rest between each exercise.

DUMBBELL SIDE LATERALS

3 sets x 20 reps with 1 chain per hand

- 30 seconds rest between each set.
- 60 seconds rest between each exercise.

INCLINE BENCH TRICEPS EXTENSION

2 sets x 30 reps with 20 lb. dumbbells

- 30 seconds rest between each set.
- 60 seconds rest between each exercise.

BOSU BALL PUSH-UP

2 sets to failure

- 60 seconds rest between sets.

TANK TOP WORKOUT #2

This workout focuses on the most important part of strength development – the infrastructure. Here we are performing exercises that will cause our much smaller stability muscles to be taxed and built stronger.

TWO-ARM BENT-OVER ROWS

1 set x 50 reps with 25 lb. dumbbells

- 60 seconds rest between each exercise.

DUMBBELL PUSH-UP

4 sets x 25 reps

- 30 seconds rest between sets.
- 60 seconds rest before new exercise.

BOSU BALL PUSH-UP

3 sets x 12 reps with bodyweight

- 30 seconds rest between sets.
- 60 seconds rest before new exercise.

CLOSE-GRIP BOSU BALL PUSH-UP

2 sets x 12 reps with bodyweight

- 30 seconds rest between sets.
- 60 seconds rest before new exercise.

CHAIN SIDE LATERALS

2 sets x 20 reps with 1 chain per side

- 30 seconds rest between sets.
- 60 seconds rest before new exercise.

TWO-ARM BENT-OVER ROWS

- 1 set x 50 reps with 25 lb. dumbbells

LOWER BODY WORKOUT #1

This is a fantastic workout to develop the powerful muscles of the lower body including the glutes, quads, hamstrings, calves and even abs. If toning and shaping are your goals, emphasize strict, slow form using just your body weight. If explosive athletic performance is your goal, emphasize forceful contractions and controlled downward motion.

PRONE PLANK

5 sets x 30 second hold

- 30 seconds rest between each set.
- 60 seconds rest between each exercise.

SINGLE LEG SPRINTER SQUAT

4 sets x 15 reps (each leg)

- 60 seconds rest between each set.
- 60 seconds rest between each exercise.

HIGH BOX STEP-UPS

2 sets x 25 reps (each leg)

- 60 seconds rest between each set.
- 60 seconds rest between each exercise.

SINGLE LEG DUMBBELL DEADLIFT

2 sets x 25 reps (each leg)

- 30 seconds rest between each set.
- 60 seconds rest between each exercise.

SIDE PLANK

5 sets x 30 seconds (each side)

- 30 seconds rest between each set.

LOWER BODY WORKOUT #2

ELBOW-TO-KNEE BACK EXTENSION

3 sets x 10 reps (Each side: left arm with right leg & right arm with left leg)

- 15 seconds rest between each movement.
- 60 seconds rest before next exercise.

HIGH-HIP BARBELL DEADLIFT

95 x 10 / 135 x 10 / 185 x 10 / 225 x 5 / 275 x 5 / 315 x 2 / 345 x 2

- 30 seconds rest between each set.
- 60 seconds rest before next exercise.

POWER SQUAT

5 sets x 8 reps with 50 lb. dumbbells

- 30 seconds rest between each set.
- 60 seconds rest before next exercise.

SINGLE LEG BENCH SQUAT

3 sets x 10 reps (each side)

- 30 seconds rest between each set.
- 60 seconds rest before next exercise.

HIGH-HIP DUMBBELL DEADLIFT

3 sets x 15 reps with 50 lb. dumbbells

- 30 seconds rest between each set.
- 60 seconds rest before next exercise.

SIDE PLANK

- 3 sets x 30 seconds (each side)
- 30 seconds rest between each set.

POWER DEADLIFT WORKOUT

This is a bread-and-butter workout for any serious athlete. If you want to add lean muscle, then this is the routine to follow. On this day, work up to your max 3-rep set. Once you can do 3 reps successfully, add 5% to the bar on your next workout. For example, today you finish with a 300 lb. deadlift for three reps. Next time, you attempt 3 reps at 315 lbs.

CHIN-UPS

3 sets x 10 reps with bodyweight

- 15 seconds rest between each set.
- 60 seconds rest before next exercise.

CONVENTIONAL BARBELL DEADLIFT

185 x 3 / 225 x 3 / 275 x 3 / 315 x 3 / 365 x 3 / 405 x 1

- 60 seconds rest between each set.
- 60 seconds rest before next exercise.

POWER SQUAT

5 sets x 5 reps with 50 lb. dumbbells

- 45 seconds rest between each set.
- 60 seconds rest before next exercise.

CONVENTIONAL DUMBBELL DEADLIFT

5 sets x 10 reps

- 30 seconds rest between each set.
- 60 seconds rest before next exercise.

GAMER TWIST

5 sets x 10 reps

- 30 seconds rest between each set.

PUSH-PULL WORKOUTS

I prefer to think in terms of motions and not muscles. If I perform a deadlift, I am training my pull muscles; hamstrings, lower back, glutes, upper back and traps. Sometimes, it makes sense to train these muscle groups together. The same holds true for the push muscles of the chest, delts, triceps, quads and calves. This workout is appropriate for novices, women, health-minded individuals and professional athletes.

PUSH WORKOUT

OVERHEAD SQUAT

5 sets x 10 reps

- 60 seconds rest between sets.
- 60 seconds rest between exercises.

INCLINE DUMBBELL PRESS

40 x 20 / 50 x 15 / 60 x 10 / 65 x 10 / 70 x 10

- 20 seconds rest between sets.
- 45 seconds rest between exercises.

DUMBBELL FRONT LATERALS

3 sets x 15 reps with 15 lb. dumbbells

- 20 seconds rest between sets.
- 45 seconds rest between exercises.

CLOSE-GRIP BOSU BALL PUSH-UP

5 sets x 10 reps

- 20 seconds rest between sets.
- 45 seconds rest between exercises.

X-PATTERN TOE TOUCH

2 sets x 50 reps (each side)

- 30 seconds rest between each set.

PULL WORKOUT

TWO-ARM BENT-OVER DUMBBELL ROW

5 sets x 8 reps

- 60 seconds rest between sets.
- 60 seconds rest before next exercise.

HIGH-HIP BARBELL DEADLIFT

135 x 20 / 185 x 10 / 225 x 5 / 275 x 3 / 315 x 2 / 365 x 1 / 385 x 1 / 405 x 1

- 60 seconds rest between sets.
- Practice deep breathing between each set.
- Rest 60 seconds before next exercise

SINGLE LEG DUMBBELL DEADLIFT

3 sets x 10 reps with 40 lb. dumbbell

- 60 seconds rest between sets.
- 60 seconds rest before next exercise.

BARBELL UPRIGHT ROW

3 sets x 15 reps with 65 lbs. (empty barbell with 10 lbs. on each side)

- 60 seconds rest between sets.
- Alternate Straight-leg Crunch
- 5 sets x 20 reps (each side)
- 30 seconds rest between each set.

CHAPTER THIRTEEN

CARDIOVASCULAR TRAINING

Cardiovascular exercise is essential to *Living Lean*. A person should incorporate 30 to 60 minutes of dedicated cardiovascular exercise three to five times a week. I prefer the treadmill for maximum effect. A few common forms of cardio are walking, running, swimming, cycling, rowing, basketball, soccer, or even Frisbee. The point is to raise your heart rate and keep it elevated for a predetermined amount of time that is relative to your medical history and training background.

The best way to begin cardio training is to walk out of your front door, down the street, touch the mailbox on the corner and walk back. The next day, walk to that same mailbox and jog back. Continue to increase your volume and/or intensity with each session. As long as you are improving on the session before, you are making progress!

If you have access to a treadmill, the following workouts are for you. If not, these principles can be applied to the elliptical, Stair Master, Precor, rowing machine, or stationary bike. You can even use your watch or cell phone timer on any street, track or trail in your neighborhood.

BEGINNER TREADMILL WORKOUT

Warm-up

- 5 minute walk at 3 mph

Round 1

- 30 second jog at 5 mph
- 2 minute walk at 3 mph

Round 2

- 30 second jog at 5 mph
- 2 minute walk at 3 mph

Round 3

- 30 second jog at 5 mph
- 2 minute walk at 3 mph

Round 4

- 30 second jog at 5 mph
- 2 minute walk at 3 mph

Cool-down

- 5 minute walk at 3 mph

GOAL: Work up to eight rounds.

HIGH INTENSITY INTERVAL TRAINING

Warm-up

- 5 minute walk at 3 mph

Round 1

- 1 minute at 8 mph
- 1 minute at 6 mph

Round 2

- 1 minute at 8 mph
- 1 minute at 6 mph

Round 3

- 1 minute at 8 mph
- 1 minute at 6 mph

Round 4

- 1 minute at 8 mph
- 1 minute at 6 mph

Round 5

- 1 minute at 8 mph
- 1 minute at 6 mph

Cool-down

- 5 minute walk at 3 mph

GOAL: Increase the speed of your sprints.

THE FIGHTER'S TREADMILL WORKOUT

Warm-up

- 5 minute walk at 3 mph

Round 1

- 1 minute at 8 mph
- 1 minute at 6 mph
- 1 minute at 8 mph
- 1 minute at 6 mph
- 1 minute at 8 mph
- 1 minute walk at 3 mph

Round 2

- 1 minute at 9 mph
- 1 minute at 6 mph
- 1 minute at 9 mph
- 1 minute at 6 mph
- 1 minute at 9 mph
- 1 minute walk at 3 mph

Round 3

- 1 minute at 10 mph
- 1 minute at 6 mph
- 1 minute at 10 mph
- 1 minute at 6 mph
- 1 minute at 10 mph

Cool-down

- 5 minute walk at 3 mph

GOAL: All three rounds at 10 mph during sprint interval.

CHAPTER FOURTEEN

Exercises

CORE

ALTERNATING STRAIGHT-LEG CRUNCH

Starting Position

- Lie flat on your back with your left heel against your glute and left knee pointing
  to the sky.
- Left hand is gently holding your neck.
- Hold right leg straight with right heel 6 inches off ground.

Action

- Contract through your abdominal wall and bring your left elbow to meet your right knee just above your sternum.
- Pause briefly for mild contraction.
- Extend to starting position.

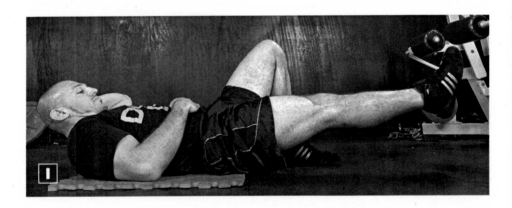

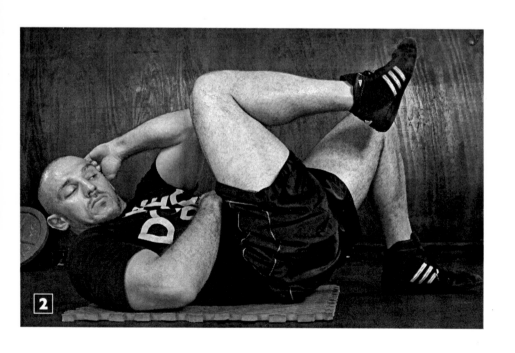

BOSU BALL SUPERMAN ALTERNATE SIDE RAISE

Starting Position

- Lie belly down on the soft part of a Bosu Ball (you can also use a Swiss ball). Make sure your hip bones and belly button are in firm contact.
- Stretch your arms long in front of you, knuckles up, with palms resting on the floor.
- Stretch your legs long behind you, with your toes resting on the floor.

Action

- Keeping your head relaxed but fixed, raise your left arm and left leg, leading with the knuckles and heel.
- Pause slightly at the top, ensuring a mild contraction across your lower back before gently lowering.
- Repeat on the opposite side, right arm and right leg.

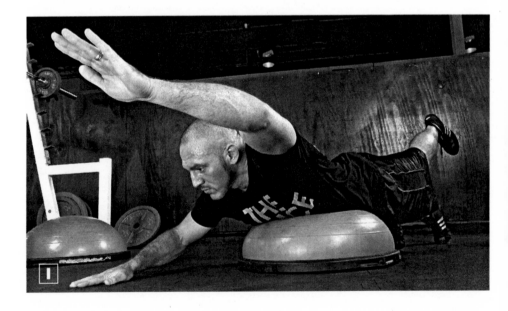

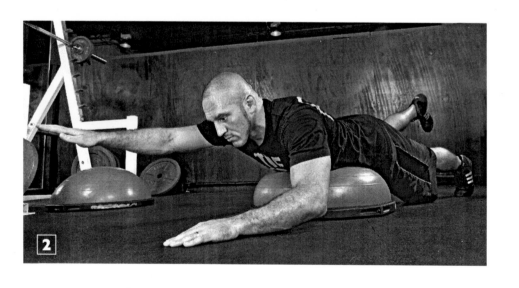

LEG RAISE DOUBLE

Starting Position

- Lie with your back flat on the ground.
- Place hands at your sides with your legs fully extended.

Action

- Raise both legs straight up off of the ground until they are perpendicular to the floor.
- Gently contract abs before smoothly lowering to starting position.

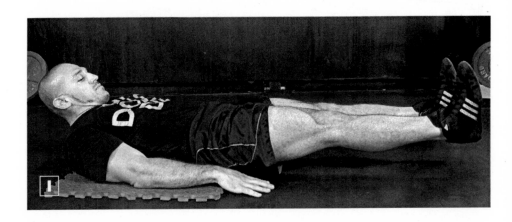

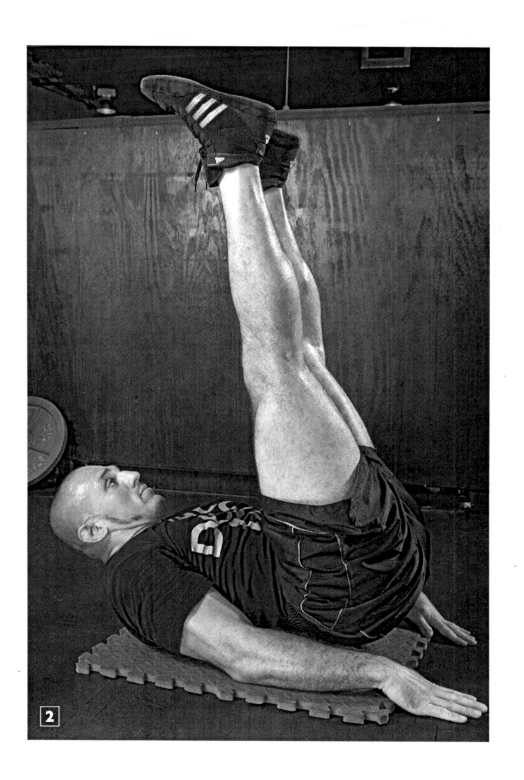

ELBOW-TO-KNEE BACK EXTENSION

Starting Position

- Assume a position on all fours, making contact with the palms of the hands, knees and toes.
- Keep your back perfectly flat by maintaining hip and shoulder stability.
- Bring your left knee and right elbow together, touching at your chest.

Action

- Simultaneously stretch your arm long in front of you while stretching your leg long behind you.
- Pause slightly at the top.
- Maintain balance while squeezing for a mild contraction across your glutes, upper hamstrings and lower back before gently lowering.

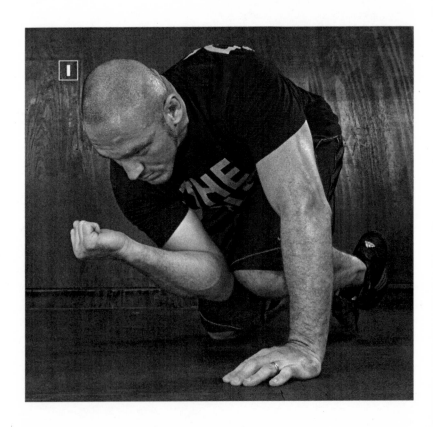

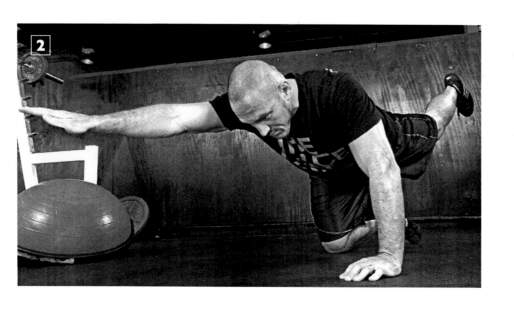

PRONE PLANK

Starting Position

- This position begins similar to a Push-up except your weight is resting on your elbows instead of your palms (see picture).

Action

- Maintain a flat back and straight legs while keeping your mid-section tight.
- Hold this position while keeping the body perfectly still.

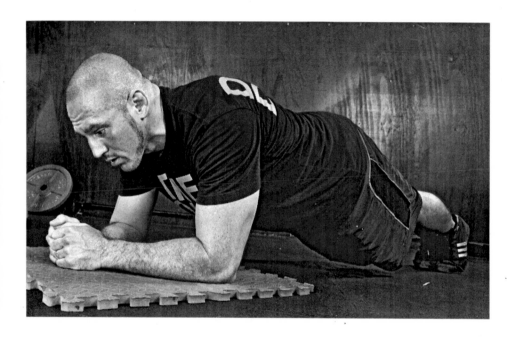

GAMER TWIST

Starting Position

- Sitting on the floor, lean back until your torso is at 45 degree angle to the ground.
- Extend your legs for balance with knees slightly bent.

Action

- Holding a dumbbell 6 inches above your chest, twist to the right.
- Pause.
- Twist to the left.
- Repeat.

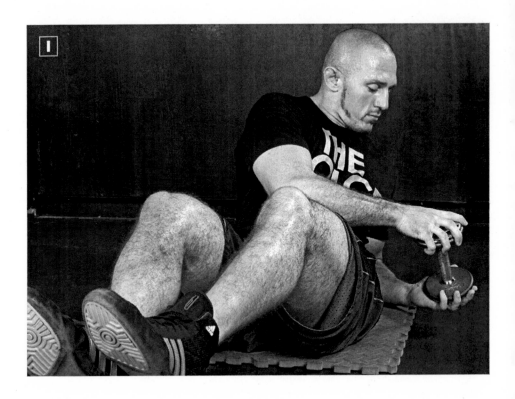

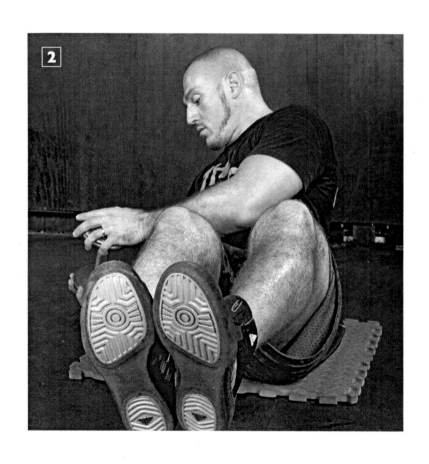

SIDE PLANK

Position

- Lie on your side.
- Rise up on elbow with knees and hip off the floor. Elbow should be at a 90 degree angle.
- Keep the spine neutral and align the head with the torso.

Action

- Hold the position until failure or for the desired duration.

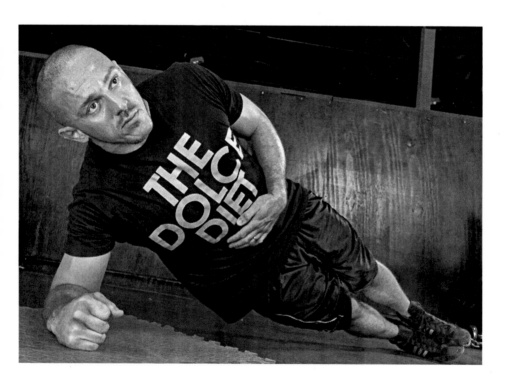

LYING TOE TOUCH

Starting Position

- Lie on your back with both legs pointed directly upward.

Action

- Roll your torso upward until your fingertips touch your toes, keeping legs straight.
- Slowly lower back down and repeat.

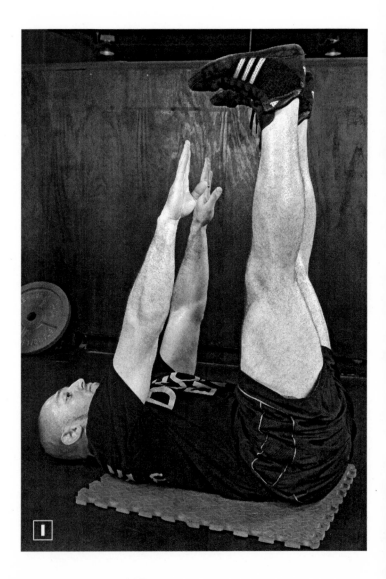

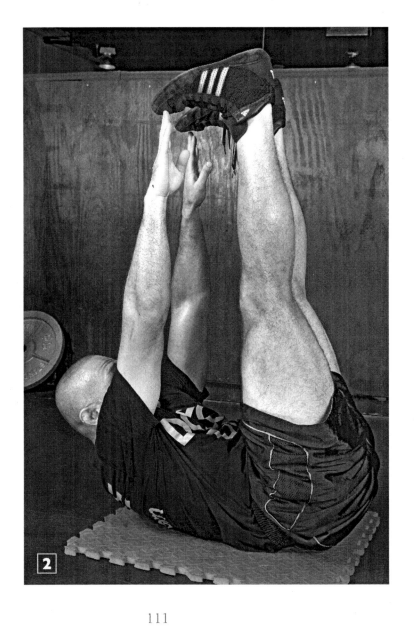

X-PATTERN TOE TOUCH

Starting Position

- Lie flat on your back with your left heel against your glute and left knee pointing to the sky.
- Left hand is extended at a 45 degree angle to your body.
- Right leg is held straight with right heel 6 inches off ground.

Action

- Contract through your abdominal wall and raise your left arm and right leg together in a fluid motion. Reach to tap your instep over your left hip.
- Pause briefly for mild contraction, slightly raising tail bone further off the floor.
- Lower to starting position.

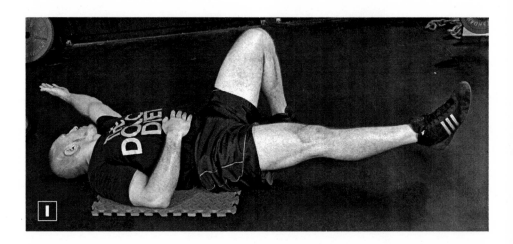

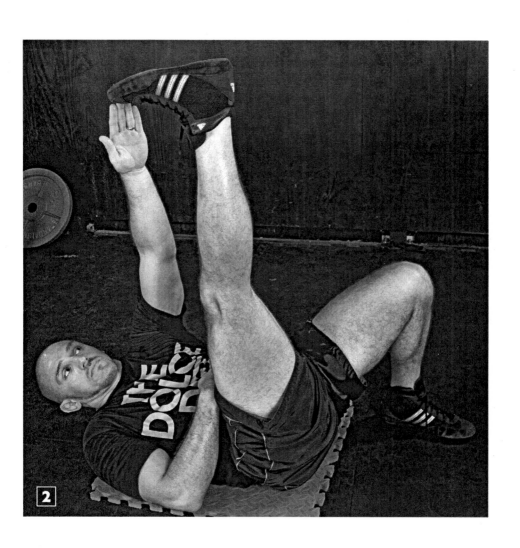

DEADLIFTS

CONVENTIONAL BARBELL DEADLIFT

Starting Position

- Stand in front of a barbell in a neutral stance: heels under knees, knees under hips and hips under shoulders.
- Look up and ease your hips backward, initiating a squat position.
- Allow your arms to hang naturally while gently reaching for the barbell.
- The barbell should be positioned mid-shoelace.

Action

- When your hips have reached near parallel to the floor, grasp the bar, just outside of your shins.
- Squeeze the bar tightly.
- Forcefully push through the floor and stand up, throwing your head backward and your hips forward.
- Return to the starting position, letting the weight settle on the floor before starting your next rep.

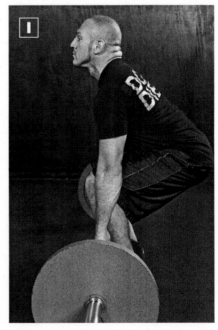

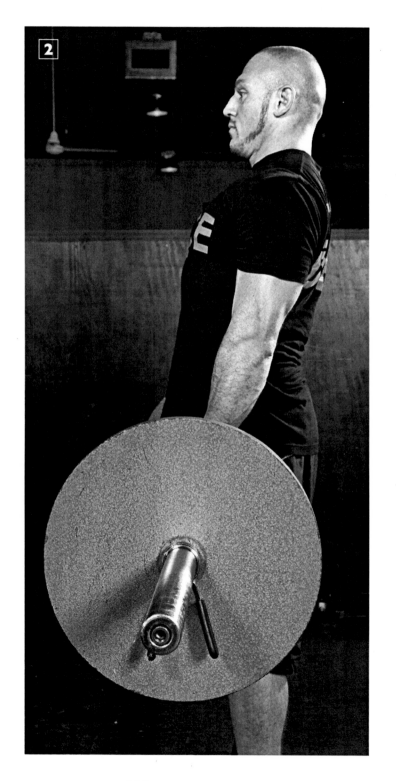

CONVENTIONAL DUMBBELL DEADLIFT

Starting Position

- Place a pair of dumbbells in front of your toes and assume a neutral stance: heels under knees, knees under hips and hips under shoulders.
- Look up and ease your hips backward, initiating a squat position.
- Allow your arms to hang naturally and gently reach for the dumbbells.

Action

- When your hips have reached near parallel to the floor, grasp the dumbbells tightly.
- Forcefully push through the floor and stand up, throwing your head backward and your hips forward.
- Return to the starting position, letting the weight settle on the floor before starting your next rep.

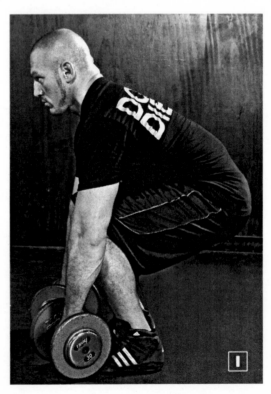

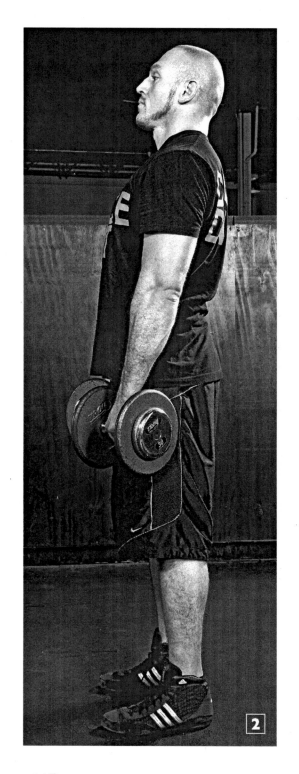

HIGH-HIP BARBELL DEADLIFT

Starting Position

- Stand in front of a barbell in a neutral stance: heels under knees, knees under hips and hips under shoulders.
- Slightly bend your knees and keep this position fixed throughout the movement.
- Looking down, the barbell should be the same distance from your shin bone as it is from the tip of your toes, approximately mid-shoelace.

Action

- Press your hips slightly backward and shift your weight onto your heels. Be sure to look straight forward and not at the floor.
- Slowly lower torso until your hands are able to grasp the bar, just outside of your shins, keeping your hips above parallel to the floor, with knees bent greater than 90 degrees.
- Squeeze the bar tightly
- Forcefully stand up, throwing your head backward and your hips forward.
- Control the weight for a pause.
- Return to the starting position, letting the weight settle on the floor before starting your next rep.

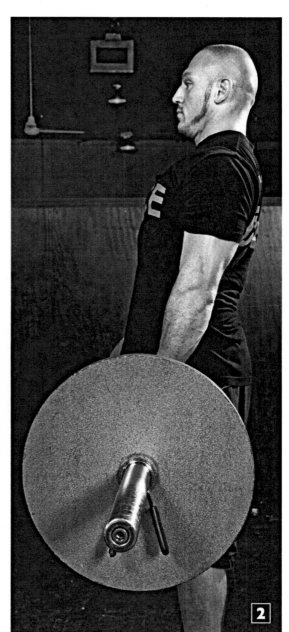

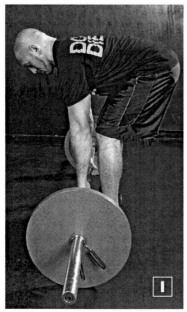

HIGH-HIP DUMBBELL DEADLIFT

Starting Position

- Place a pair of dumbbells in front of your toes while standing in a neutral stance: heels under knees, knees under hips and hips under shoulders.
- Looking forward, ease your hips backward and lean your torso forward.
- Allow your arms to hang naturally, gently reaching for the dumbbells.

Action

- Grasp the dumbbells, keeping your hips above parallel to the floor.
- Forcefully stand up, throwing your head backward and your hips forward.
- Control the weight for a pause.
- Return to the starting position.
- Let weight settle on the floor before starting your next rep.

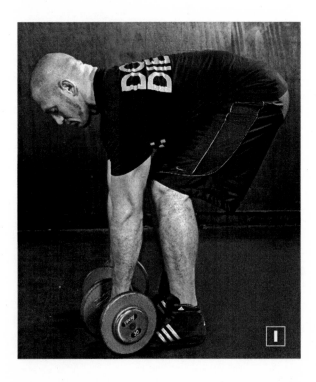

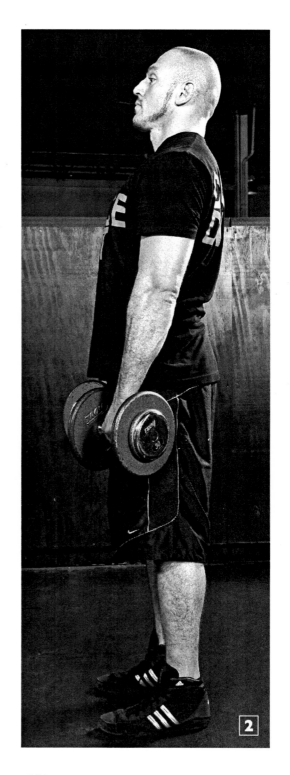

SINGLE LEG DUMBBELL DEADLIFT

Starting Position

- Stand on one leg and hold a dumbbell in the opposite hand.
- Keep your non-post leg gently raised behind you.

Action

- Push back your hips and lower the dumbbell to touch the floor in front of your post leg while keeping your back flat.
- Use your opposite hand for balance.
- Straighten and raise your non-post leg behind you.
- Pause slightly at bottom before returning to the starting position.

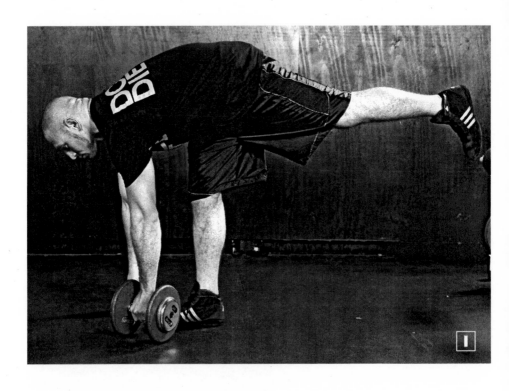

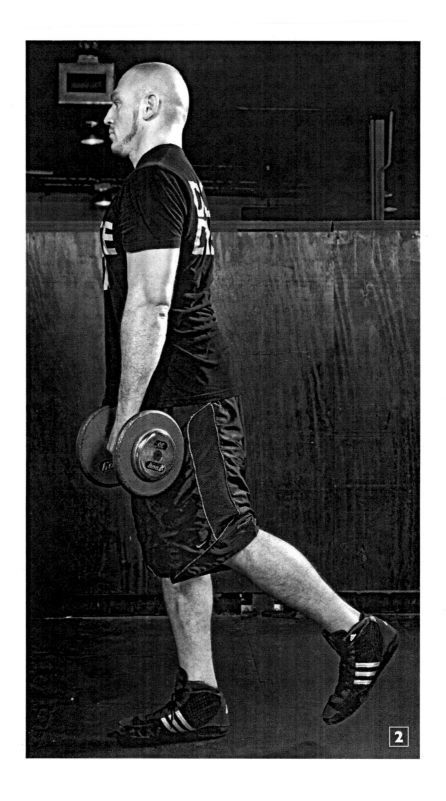

LATERALS

CHAIN SIDE LATERALS

Starting Position

- Assume a neutral stance.
- Grab the end links of each chain, allowing the chain to gather just outside of your feet.

Action

- In a fluid arc, raise each chain out to your side, finishing as your hand is parallel to your shoulder.
- Pause briefly at the top.
- Lower the chain in a controlled fashion.

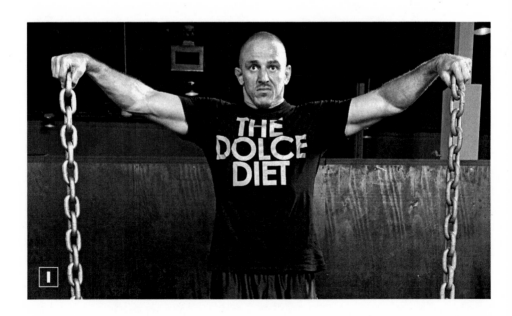

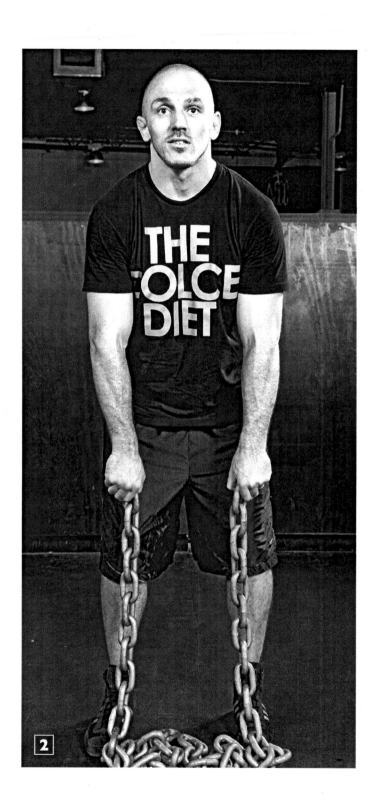

DUMBBELL FRONT LATERALS

Starting Position

- Stand with feet slightly wider than shoulder-width apart.
- Grasp a pair of dumbbells and allow them to rest naturally on your thighs.
- Keep your head up, back flat and look forward.

Action

- Raise dumbbells by leading with your thumbs.
- Bring them together at a point just above your eyes.
- Pause for mild contraction.
- Lower to a point just wider than your hips.

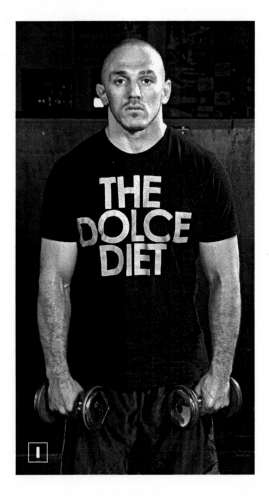

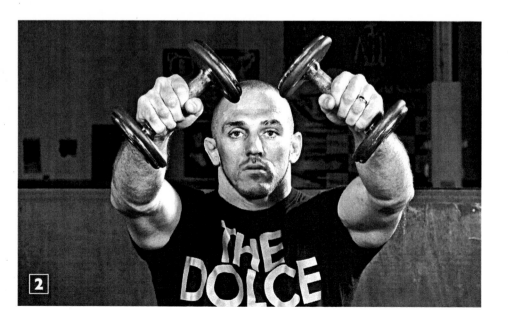

DUMBBELL SIDE LATERALS

Starting Position

- Stand with feet slightly wider than shoulder-width apart.
- Grasp a pair of dumbbells and allow to rest naturally, at arm's length, against the thighs.
- Keep head up, back flat and look forward.

Action

- Raise both dumbbells out to the side simultaneously.
- Tilt the rear of the dumbbell slightly upward at the top of the motion.
- Pause for mild contraction.
- Gently lower to starting position.

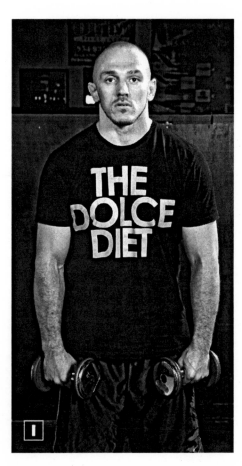

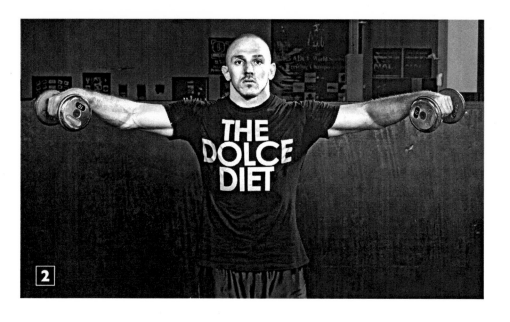

LUNGES

BACKWARD DUMBBELL LUNGE

Starting Position

- Standing with feet shoulder-width apart, grasp a dumbbell in each hand.
- Look forward with chest held high and shoulders back.

Action

- Take a step backwards and slowly lower your weight until both knees are at 90 degree angles.
- Do not rest knee on floor.
- Using your front leg, press yourself back to starting position.

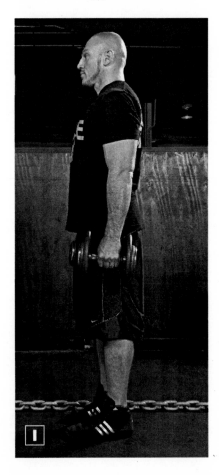

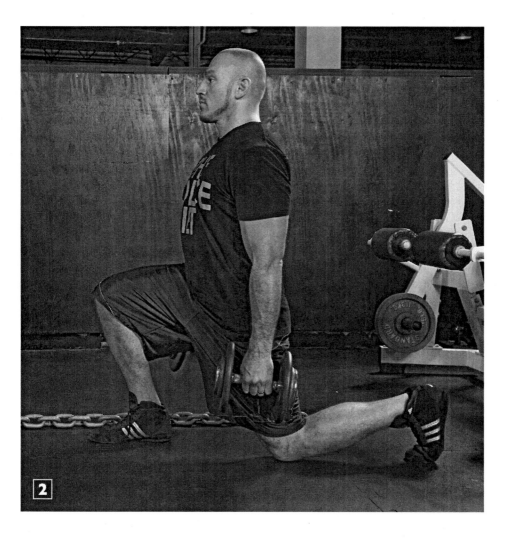

FORWARD DUMBBELL LUNGE

Starting Position

- Standing with feet shoulder-width apart, grasp a dumbbell in each hand.
- Look forward with chest held high and shoulders back.

Action

- Take a step forward and slowly lower your weight until both knees are at 90 degree angles.
- Do not rest knee on floor.
- Using your front leg, press yourself back to starting position.

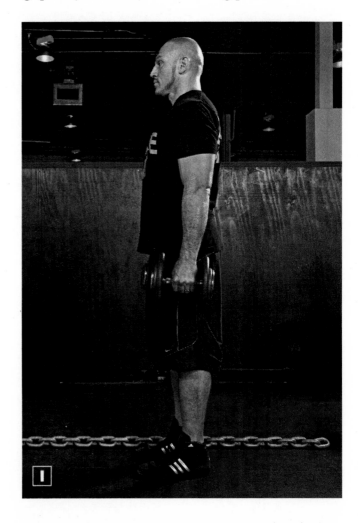

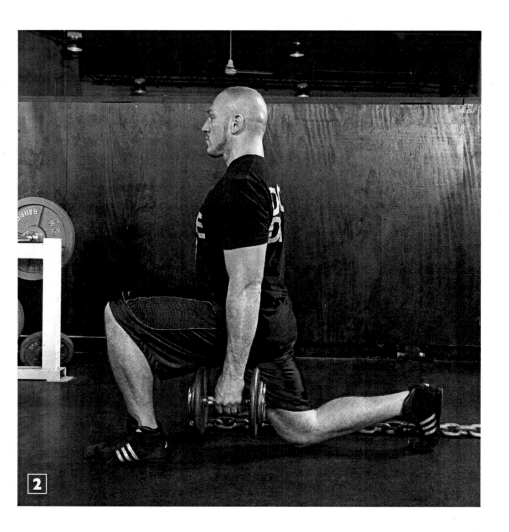

PRESSES

BARBELL BENCH PRESS

Starting Position

- Lay on the bench, making sure to evenly distribute your weight amongst your feet, glutes, shoulders and head. This is your foundation.
- Grasp the bar at even points about 6 inches wider than your shoulders.
- Remove the bar from the upright rack by extending at the elbows and pushing your torso deeply into the bench.

Action

- Maintaining your foundation, gently rotate your elbows inward, take in a deep breath and lower the bar in a controlled motion until it touches your lower chest.
- Press the barbell upwards to the starting position with a slight arc towards your head.

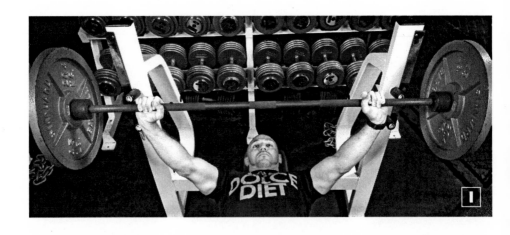

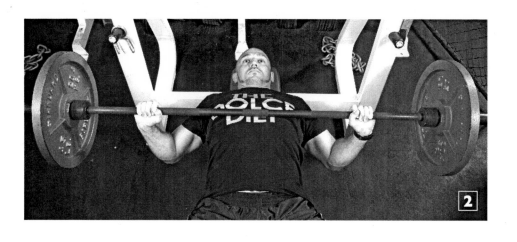

INCLINE BENCH TRICEPS EXTENSION

Starting Position

- Set the bench at a 45 degree angle to the floor.
- Lay back on the bench making sure your head extends above the top of the seat by standing on the floor or squatting on the bench (see picture).
- Extend dumbbells to full extension.

Action

- Lower the dumbbells past your head, keeping your elbows pointed toward the ceiling.
- Smoothly raise dumbbells back to starting point.

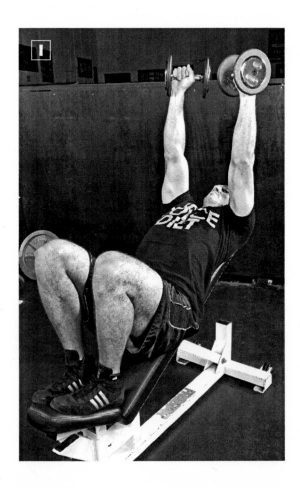

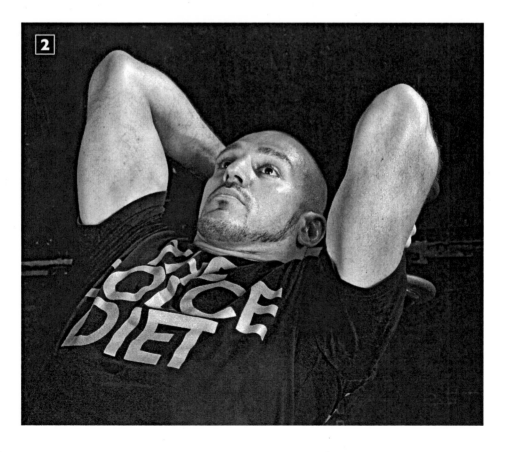

INCLINE DUMBBELL PRESS

Starting Position

- Set the bench at a 45 degree angle to the floor.
- Grasp the dumbbells and set on your thighs as you sit back.
- Using the strength of your legs, raise each dumbbell to the starting position (see picture).

Action

- Take in a deep breath and lower the dumbbells in a controlled motion until your upper arms are parallel with the floor.
- Smoothly press the dumbbells upwards to the starting position.

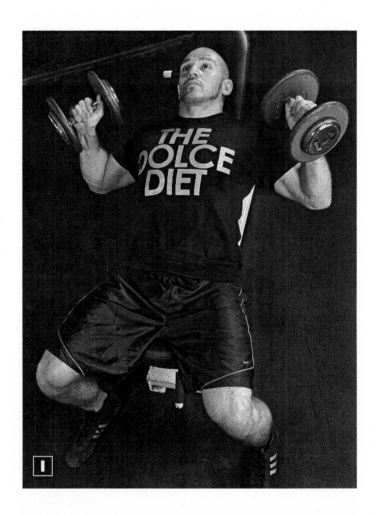

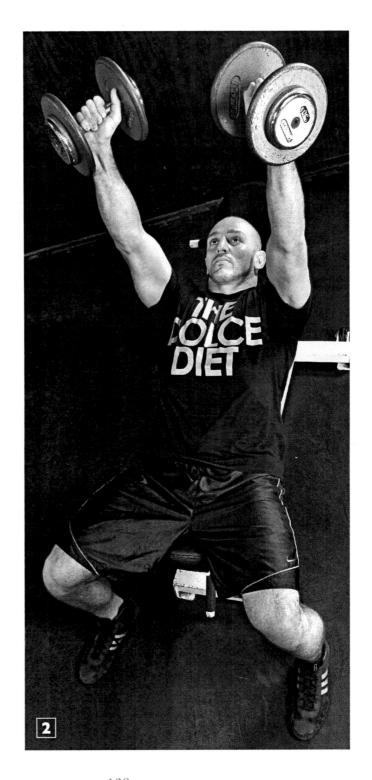

PUSH-UPS

PUSH-UP

Starting Position

- Lie face down with your legs straight and toes in contact with the floor.
- Place the palm of your hands on the floor just outside of your chest.

Action

- Keeping a flat back and tight mid-section, press your torso upwards until arms are completely extended.
- Lower until upper arms are parallel with floor before pressing back up.

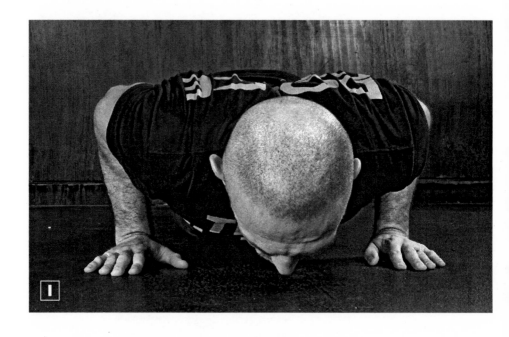

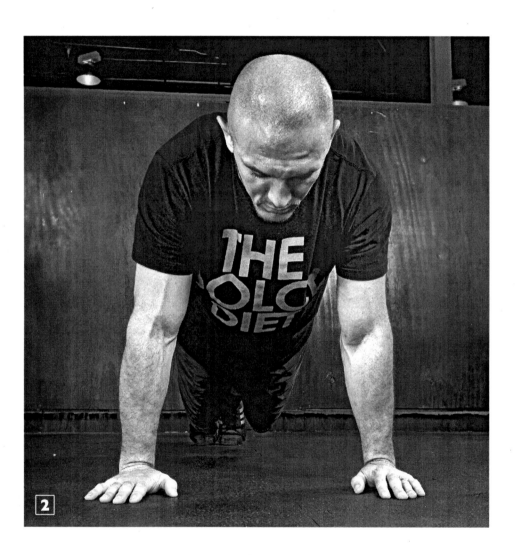

CHAIN PUSH-UP

- Perform this exercise exactly as the standard Push-up with the addition of a chain over your shoulder.

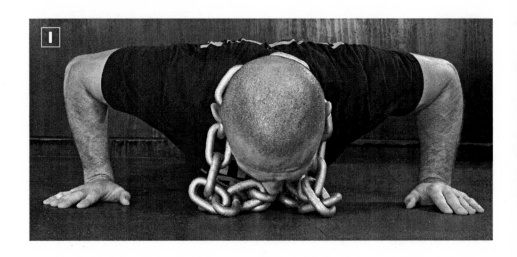

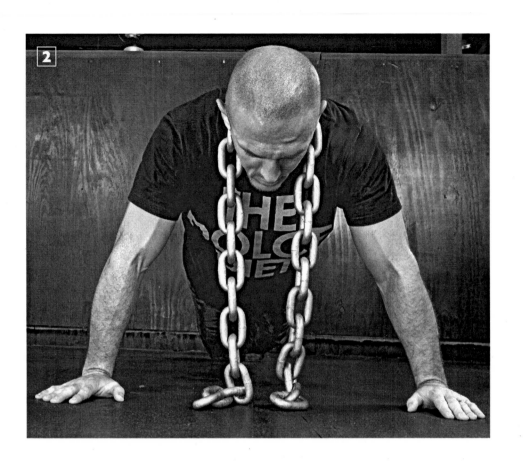

DUMBBELL PUSH-UP

- Perform this exercise exactly as the standard Push-up with the addition of a dumbbell in each hand to increase range of motion.

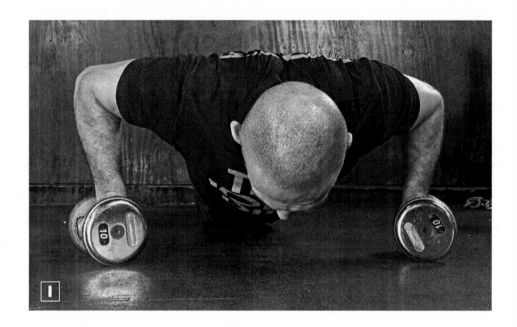

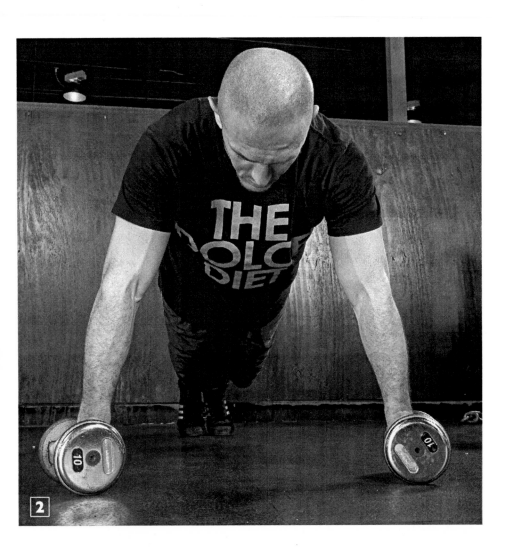

BOSU BALL PUSH-UP

Starting Position

- Place a Bosu Ball on the floor, with the round side down.
- Grab the outer edge of the platform.
- Position your legs as you would in a standard Push-up position.

Action

- Lower your torso until your chest touches the platform.
- Forcefully press yourself back to the starting position.
- Work to maintain balance at all times.

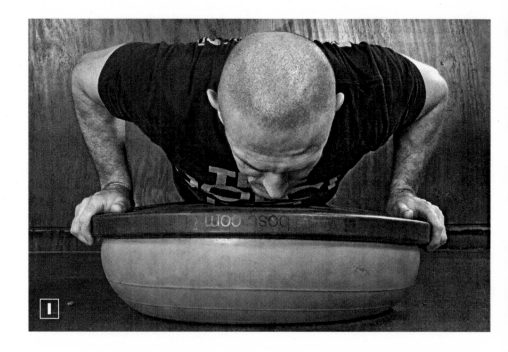

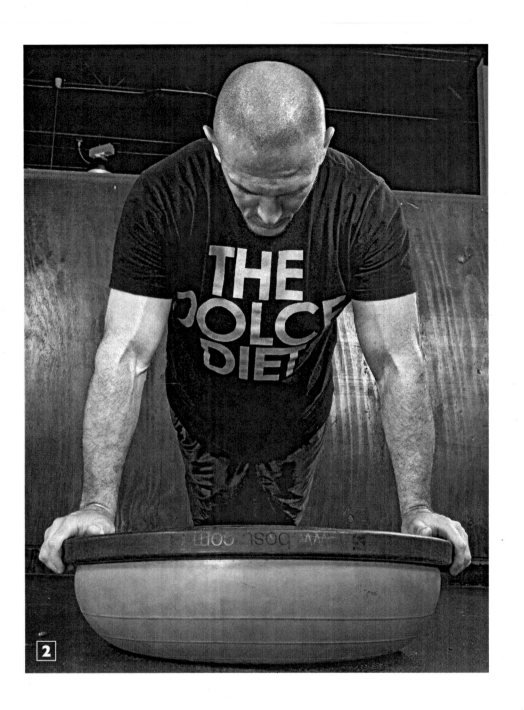

CLOSE GRIP BOSU BALL PUSH-UP

Starting Position

- Place a Bosu Ball on the floor, with flat side down.
- Position your hands in the middle of the ball, 4-6 inches apart.
- Position your legs as you would in a standard Push-up position.

Action

- Lower your torso until your chest touches your hands.
- Forcefully press back to the starting position.
- Work to maintain balance at all times.

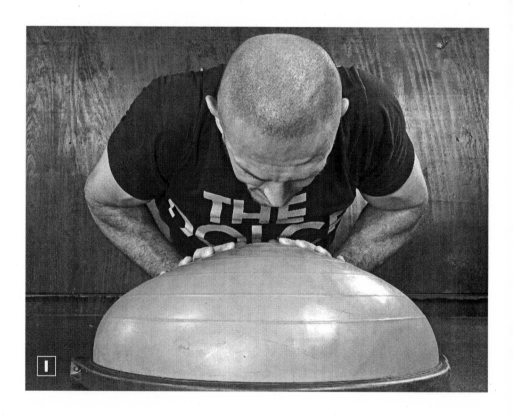

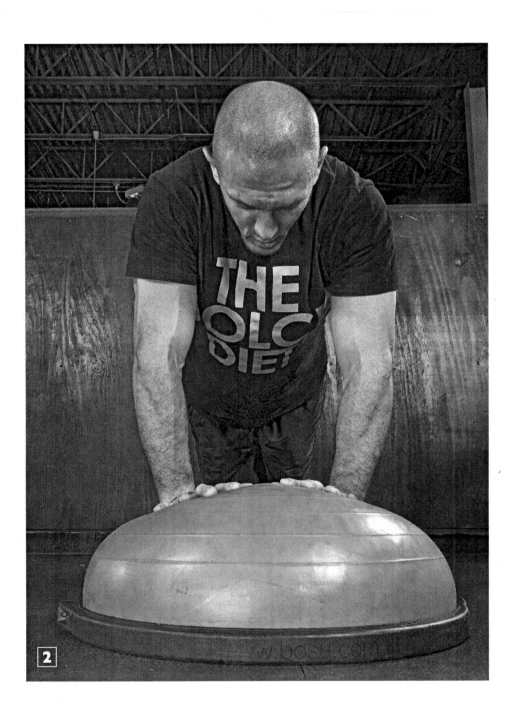

ROWS

BARBELL UPRIGHT ROW

Starting Position

- Stand upright and take a narrow grip on the barbell with hands approximately 6-12 inches apart.

Action

- Keep the barbell close to the body and pull, leading with the elbows, until the bar reaches your upper chest/chin.
- Pause slightly at the top.
- Lower slowly to starting position while maintaining full control.

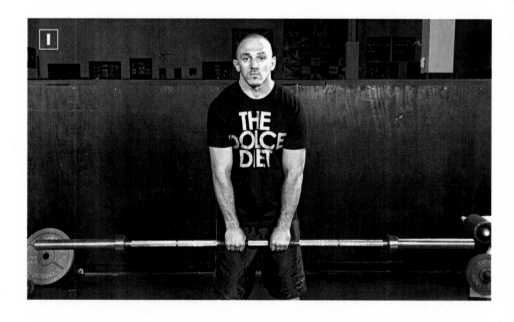

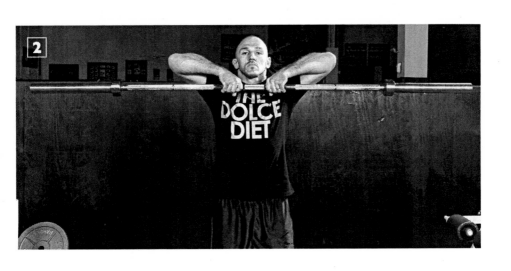

BENT-OVER TWO-ARM DUMBBELL ROW

Starting Position

- Grasp each dumbbell with palms facing inward and stand tall.
- Keeping your feet shoulder width apart, bend your knees slightly and push your hips backward until your torso is parallel to the floor.

Action

- While keeping the torso stationary and back flat, pull the dumbbells to your "pants pockets," keeping your elbows tucked in.
- Pause for a brief contraction before slowly lowering the weight again to the starting position.
- Maintain control of the weight throughout each repetition.

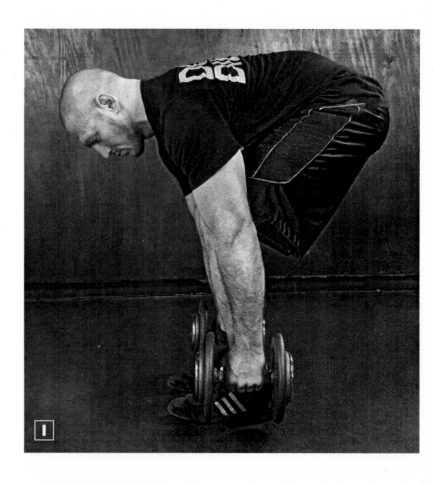

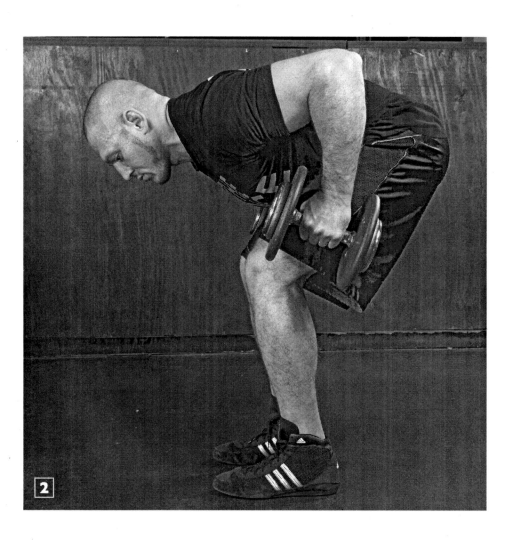

SQUATS

HIGH BOX STEP-UPS

Starting Position

- Step one foot on a box, bench or platform at a height between 12 and 36 inches.
- Look forward with head held high.

Action

- Through your heel, forcefully push off the box and stand at an upright position.
- Kick the non-working leg backward, leading with the heel and mildly contracting the glute.
- Slowly control the descent and repeat.

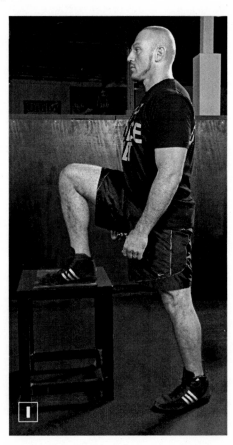

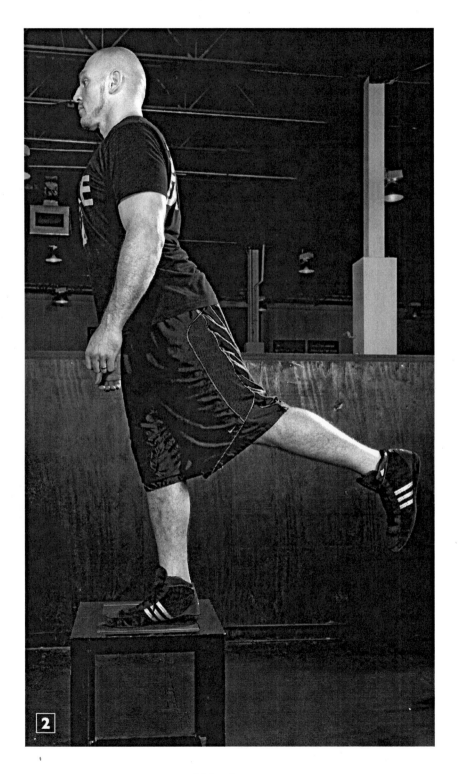

POWER SQUAT

Starting Position

- Stand with dumbbells grasped to sides.
- Clean dumbbells up to shoulders so side of each dumbbell rests on top of each shoulder.
- Balance dumbbells on shoulders.

Action

- Bend knees forward while allowing hips to bend back behind, keeping back straight and knees pointed same direction as feet.
- Descend until thighs are just past parallel to floor.
- Extend knees and hips until legs are straight. Repeat.

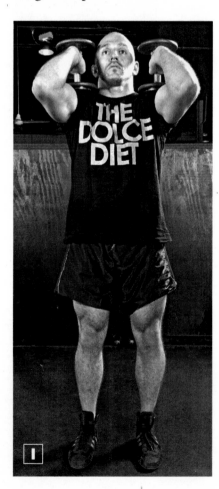

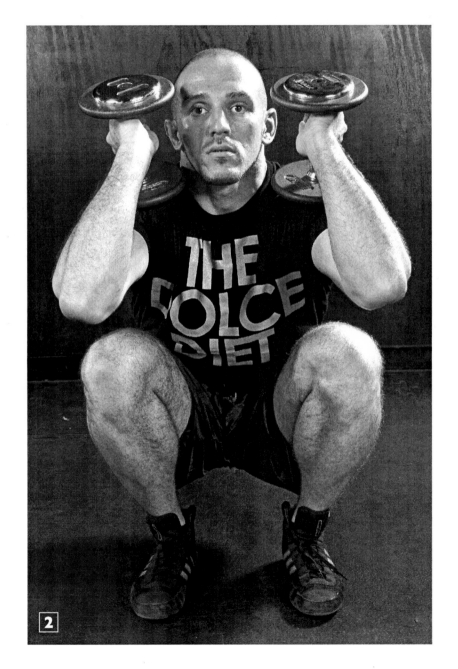

SINGLE LEG SPRINTER SQUAT

Starting Position

- Stand on one leg with your opposite leg bent at a 90 degree angle and gently hold your hands forward for balance.

Action

- Slowly lower your body in a squat motion until your rear knee can touch your opposite ankle (see picture).
- Drive through your heel and push your body to the starting position.

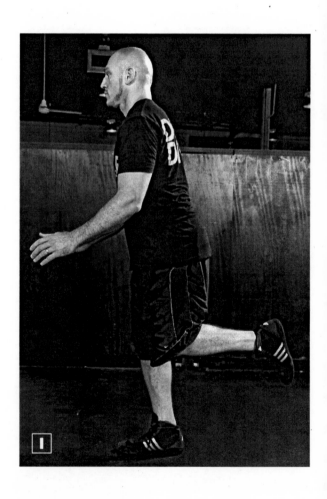

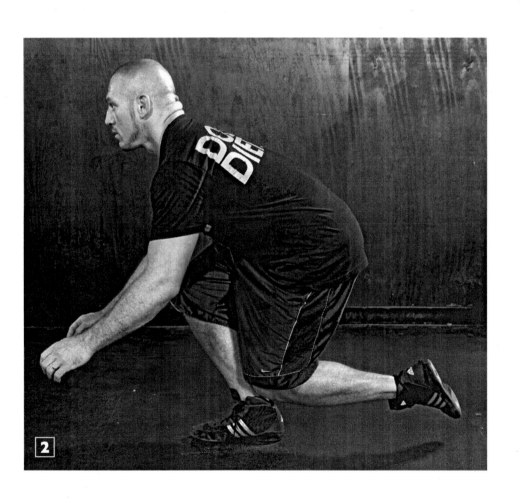

SINGLE LEG BENCH SQUAT

Starting Position

- Sit down on a standard bench.
- Firmly plant one foot on the floor.
- Extend the non-working leg as straight as possible.

Action

- Push down through your heel and forcefully stand on one leg.
- Maintain balance with your arms.
- Keep your non-working leg as high as possible.
- Slowly extend your hips backward to descend onto the bench.

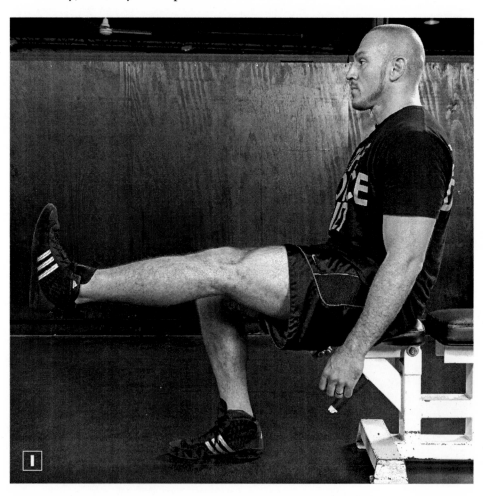

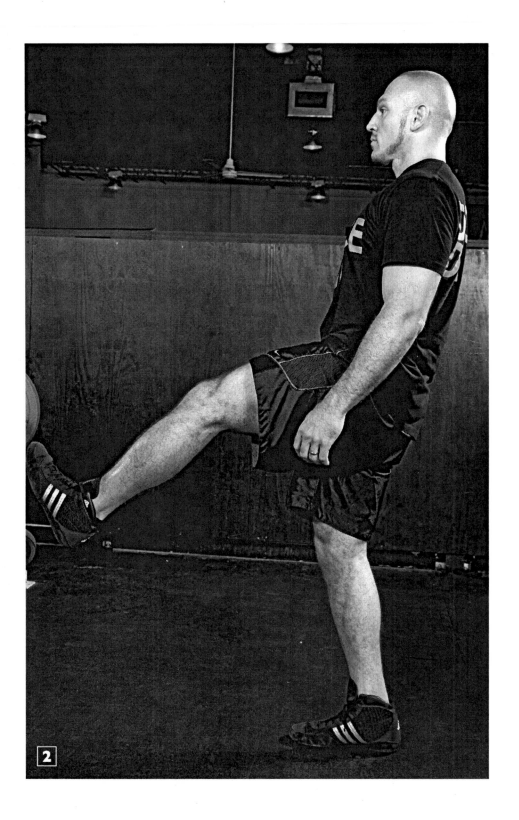

2

161

OVERHEAD SQUAT

Starting Position

- Grab one dumbbell and stand with feet slightly wider than shoulder-width apart.
- Press dumbbell above your head and allow non-working arm to hang naturally.

Action

- Look forward with your chest held high and push your hips backward to begin the descent of a squat.
- With your non-working arm, try to touch the floor, while keeping the dumbbell pressed to full extension.
- When maximum depth has been reached, push through the heels to your starting position.

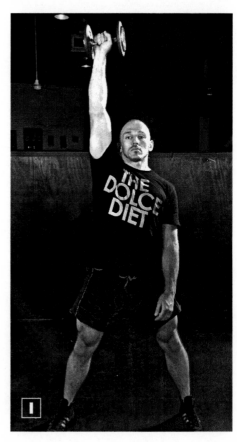

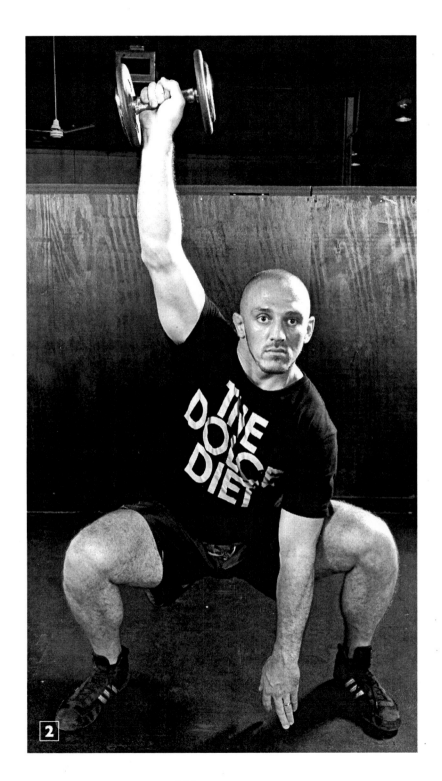

PRAISE FOR
THE DOLCE DIET:
THREE WEEKS TO SHREDDED

"Thanks to Mike Dolce, I am sitting here today at a healthy 172 lbs. after weighing in last February 1st at 340 lbs. This is a new life that I've grown into with the help of Mike and The Dolce Diet. I strongly recommend the Three Weeks to Shredded program."
—*Justin B.*

"Started at 215 lbs. back in April, now I'm 178! Thanks, Mike, for all the help and motivation."
—*David W.*

"When I started The Dolce Diet I was a 40-inch waist weighing in at 265 lbs. Six weeks later I'm a 36-inch waist and 50 lbs. lighter!"
—*Anderson W.*

"After one week on this plan, I've dropped six pounds. SIX! For a woman that has been scale-conscious the past five years that was amazing to me. I can't thank Mike enough for creating this and putting it out there for all of us to experience for ourselves. I wish this was around years ago."
—*Jennifer C.*

"I'm down another 6 lbs. That's 11 lbs. in 7 days!"
—*Imran R.*

"Working 60 hours a week but three weeks in on The Dolce Diet & I've lost 30 lbs. This is an awesome diet! Thank you so much for putting this out there for everyone!"
—*Nate F.*

"This week, I fit into a size 6, and literally cried. It was a huge moment in my life. For the past 6 years it's been a hassle getting ready in the mornings and having nothing fit and everything too tight. Barely squeezing into jeans made for one horrible day and frame of mind. But Monday morning when I fit into a pair of jeans I had from long ago, with nothing hanging over the sides, no jumping up and down to pull them up, just slipping into these cute pair of jeans that I've kept in the closet for motivation was a damn good feeling."
—Lyndsey F.

"The Dolce Diet is well worth it! I lost 10 lbs. in a week. This is the lightest I've been since high school!"
—Justin A.

"I've lost over 75 lbs. (and counting) as a student of Mike Dolce's. I have a second chance to live my life!"
—Bonnie W.

"14 lbs. gone in 14 days on The Dolce Diet!"
—Jason L.

"Mike and his Dolce Diet transformed me physically and mentally into who I am today. I started at 32.6% body fat & last tested at 8.7%. Thanks for everything Mike!"
—Brian S.

"I've lost 45 lbs.! I'd recommend anyone buy The Dolce Diet."
—Craig L.

"I'm down 25 lbs. in two months! People have seen my changes and are encouraged to begin their transformation."
—Mike P.

"219 lbs. to 193 in a month-and-a-half thanks to The Dolce Diet!"
—Jake C.

"The book has worked wonders already! I dropped 15+ lbs. Thanks!"
—Monroe D.

"I went from 220 lbs. to 180 in 1 month on The Dolce Diet."
—Mark A.

"Just finished my first 21-day weight cut on The Dolce Diet, and I'm in the best shape of my life! Successfully cut from 185 to 168! Thanks for doin' whatcha do!"
—John P.

"Fifteen pounds lost in 21 days! The Dolce Diet included great results, improved energy levels, more efficient training sessions and clearer thinking. Thank you, Mike Dolce, for making permanent, positive changes to my life."
—Heather P.

"In two weeks I dropped 13 lbs. and my buddy has dropped 10 lbs. Things are looking good! Thanks!"
—Andrew M.

"In 17 days I dropped over 18 lbs. I'm looking and feeling fantastic!"
—Aaron R.

"I've been doing The Dolce Diet for almost five months, and I have lost a total of 40 lbs."
—Mary, 55.

"I'm under 200 lbs. in a few weeks! I've lost just over 17 lbs. & I'm so excited about it."
—Aaron F.

"The Dolce Diet is killing me. In another two weeks I will be broke from having to replace all of my jeans and shorts with smaller sizes. I literally have lost a waist size in two weeks. Absolute truth."
—Wes H.

"Started The Dolce Diet at 209.8 lbs. It's Day 4 and I'm at 203.6 lbs.!"
—Tom C.

"80 lb. loss mark today. The Dolce Diet and determination truly goes a long way."
—Allen C.

"I lost 50lbs in about 2 months with The Dolce Diet. Mike knows what you need and he keeps it natural."
—Joseph K.

"Weighed in this morning at 143.0 lbs. Huge accomplishment for me. That's a total of 25 lbs. lost since I started The Dolce Diet. Thanks, Mike!"
—Cameron C.

"The Dolce Diet helped me lose 58 lbs. and changed my life. Thank you so much, Mike."
—Conor W.

"I was 216 and now I'm 186; almost to my goal of 170 and now I can give a shout-out to my ab muscles!"
—Eric B.

P.S. WE'D LOVE TO HEAR FROM YOU!

TWITTER
Follow Mike on Twitter @TheDolceDiet

FACEBOOK
Check out The Dolce Diet fan page at Facebook.com/
TheDolceDiet

YOUTUBE
Be sure to check out The Dolce Diet YouTube channel at
YouTube.com/dolcediet for videos detailing exercises, recipes
and so much more!

THE DOLCE DIET SOCIAL NETWORK
It's FREE! Design your own profile page at MYDolceDiet.com
and talk with Mike during his frequent LIVE CHATS, as well as
others living healthy, vibrant lifestyles just like yourself!

OFFICIAL WEBSITE
Get the latest news about Mike, his athletes, health tips and more
at TheDolceDiet.com